Popular Guide to Homeopathy

Also from Westphalia Press
westphaliapress.org

Popular Guide to Homeopathy for Family and Private Use

by Smith & Worthington

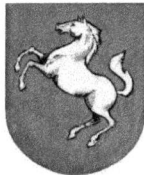

WESTPHALIA PRESS

An Imprint of Policy Studies Organization

Westphalia Press
An imprint of Policy Studies Organization
1527 New Hampshire Ave., NW
Washington, D.C. 20036
info@ipsonet.org

ISBN-13: 978-1-63391-566-4
ISBN-10: 1-63391-566-2

Cover design by Jeffrey Barnes:
jbarnesbook.design

Daniel Gutierrez-Sandoval, Executive Director
PSO and Westphalia Press

Updated material and comments on this edition
can be found at the Westphalia Press website:
www.westphaliapress.org

POPULAR GUIDE

TO

HOMŒOPATHY,

FOR

Family and Private Use:

COMPILED FROM THE STANDARD WORKS OF

PULTE, HERING, HEMPEL, AND RUDDOCK.

FOR THE USE OF

TWENTY-SEVEN HOMŒOPATHIC REMEDIES

CINCINNATI:

SMITH'S HOMŒOPATHIC PHARMACY,

No. 143 WEST FOURTH STREET.

1888.

PREFACE.

THIS Book is intended to be, as its title indicates, a guide for the treatment of simple ailments. To treat diseases with success, a knowledge of Anatomy, Physiology, Pathology, the Materia Medica, etc., is essential; and the opponents of Homœopathy allege that we ignore these sciences, because we place in the hands of unprofessional persons, ignorant of them, works on the treatment of diseases. But these objectors seem to forget that every family practices Physic more or less; it would be no easy matter to calculate the quantities of Epsom salts, pills, bitters, herbs, and patent medicines yearly employed in domestic practice, in the attempt to relieve complaints which are too trivial to call in medical assistance; and who does not know many instances where the hap-hazard administration of such medicines does infinitely more harm than good? It is to guide families in the treatment of these simple complaints, and to spread the advantages of Homœopathy, that this and similar books are published; and we would caution all laymen against attempting to treat any but simple ailments, and not even to persevere in the treatment of these, if, after a reasonable period of time, improvement does not take place. Slight indisposition is but too frequently the precursor of dangerous disease. The remedies mentioned under the heads Diphtheria, Scarlet Fever, Cholera, and other serious diseases, are only intended to be used until a Homœopathic Physician can be summoned; while such diseases require all the skill of an educated physician, valuable time, and even life itself, may frequently be saved by following the treatment laid down in the following pages.

CONTENTS.

PART I.

INTRODUCTION.

PART II.

DISEASES AND THEIR TREATMENT.

Fevers.

Eruptive Fevers.

(v)

vi   *Contents.*

Affections of the Mind.

Affections of the Head.

Affections of the Face, Eyes, Nose, and Ears.

Affections of the Teeth, Gums, and Mouth.

Affections of the Bowels.

Affections of the Skin.

x   *Contents.*

PART III.

THE MEDICINES AND THEIR USES.

PART 1.

INTRODUCTION.

LIST OF MEDICINES

Prescribed in this Book, with their English Names.

1. Aconitum napellus. — *Monkshood.*
2. Antimonium tartaricum. — *Tartar emetic.*
3. Arsenicum album. — *Arsenious acid.*
4. Belladonna. — *Deadly nightshade.*
5. Bryonia alba. — *White bryony.*
6. Calcarea carbonica. — *Carbonate of lime.*
7. Camphora. — *Camphor.*
8. Carbo vegetabilis. — *Vegetable charcoal.*
9. Chamomilla. — *Chamomile.*
10. Cinchona or China. — *Peruvian bark.*
11. Cina. — *Worm seed.*
12. Coffea cruda. — *Raw coffee.*
13. Colocynthis. — *Colocynth apple.*
14. Cuprum aceticum. — *Acetate of copper.*
15. Dulcamara. — *Bitter-sweet.*
16. Hepar sulph. calcarea. — *Sulphuret of lime.*
17. Ignatia amara. — *St. Ignatius' bean.*
18. Ipecacuanha. — *Ipecac.*

19.	Kali bichromicum.	*Bichromate of potash.*
20.	Mercurius.	*Mercury.*
21.	Nux vomica.	*Nux vomica.*
22.	Phosphorus.	*Phosphorus.*
23.	Pulsatilla.	*Meadow anemone.*
24.	Rhus toxicodendron.	*Poison oak.*
25.	Spongia tosta.	*Burnt sponge.*
26.	Sulphur.	*Sulphur.*
27.	Veratrum alb.	*White hellebore.*

EXTERNAL APPLICATIONS.

Arnica.—Mix two teaspoonfuls of the *tincture* with half a tumblerful of water, to make a lotion.

Uses.—Bruises of all kinds.

Calendula.—The lotion may be made by mixing two teaspoonfuls of the *tincture* with half a tumblerful of water.

Uses.—Cuts or lacerated wounds.

Urtica urens.—Mix one part of the *tincture* with about nine parts of water, or, still better, whisky.

Uses.—Burns and scalds.

The Dilution or strength of the medicines recommended in this work is the third potency of the vegetable and the sixth of the mineral preparations, except when otherwise directed.

The medicines may be used in the form of globules, tinctures, or dilutions. From our own experience, we should generally recommend the globules, on account of their convenience, and as we consider them equally effective, except when otherwise directed.

For adults we recommend six to ten globules, and for children from two to six globules, as a dose ; or the medicines may be administered in solution, thirty globules, six drops of dilution, or six grains of trituration, dissolved in half a tumbler of pure water, and one to two teaspoonfuls at a dose.

The globules are prepared from pure sugar of milk, which are afterward saturated with the medicinal substance in dilution or tincture.

HOW TO SELECT THE REMEDY FOR A DISEASE.

In Part III the reader will find, under each disease, the indication or signs of a medicine, which point it out as the best and most appropriate remedy to administer, because there is a more or less accurate likeness between the symptoms of the disease and those which the medicine can produce in health. That medicine, then, is always to be chosen which bears the closest analogy in its action to the symptoms which the disease manifests. For each complaint two or more medicines are mentioned, the indications of the latter being noted down to compare with the patient's sufferings.

The reader will find more copious indications of each medicine given, and, when in doubt as to the most suitable remedy, he can refer to this place, and determine the point by tracing the resemblance between the medicine's action and the disease's symptoms.

Should the symptoms of an existing disease change their character after a medicine has been given, that medicine must no longer be continued, but another substituted more suited to the new symptoms. In some cases the symptoms of a disease are either so numerous or so varied that one medicine is not sufficient to "cover" or complete the analogy of them all. In this case another may be chosen, which will include the more prominent symptoms. The two medicines are not to be mixed, for this would interfere with their respective properties and actions, but dissolved separately, and given alternately or in turns ; that is, a dose of one medicine and then a dose of the other, and so on.

MODE OF MIXING AND TAKING THE GLOBULES.

The prescribed number of globules may be placed upon the tongue, left to dissolve, and then swallowed ; but the better plan is to dissolve them in a perfectly clean tumbler, half full of pure, filtered water, or that which has been boiled and allowed to cool ; cover the tumbler, and keep it in a cool place. Use a clean spoon, which is not to be left in the medicine ; those made of porcelain are the best. A few drops of spirits of wine will keep the medicine fit for use for several days. The medicine should not, if possible, be taken during the hour before or that after a meal. *The frequency or necessary repetition of the dose* is given with every medicine in the treatment of each disease. As soon, however, as the symptoms diminish, the medicine must be given at longer intervals, and then discontinued.

With respect to "Diet," while taking the homœopathic medicines, care should be taken to avoid those articles of food possessing medicinal or stimulating properties. For this reason it is desirable to abstain from coffee, strong or green tea, acids, pickles, etc., as they are antidotes to most of the medicines, and, consequently, when partaken of, must retard the cure. Let the food, in general, be plain and nutritious; consisting of such things as are in season, simply but well cooked, without any condiments.

PART II.

DISEASES AND THEIR TREATMENT

For the Dose of the Medicines, see page XIII.

ABSCESS.

SYMPTOMS.—A collection of purulent matter in a tumor, the result of local inflammation, and which terminates in suppuration.

Belladonna, when there is much swelling, pain and inflammation. A dose three times a day.

Hepar, when matter begins to form. A dose three times a day.

Mercurius, when the abscess is shining and red, or when it is situated in the vicinity of glands. A dose three times a day.

GENERAL DIRECTIONS.—When the abscess is coming to a head, the application of a bread-and-water or linseed-

1

meal poultice will be found serviceable in promoting the suppurative process; afterward the cold water bandage may be applied as soon as the gathering has discharged freely. (See Boils, Gumboil, Whitlow, etc.)

APOPLEXY.

SYMPTOMS. — Loss of consciousness, speech and motion; face flushed or pale; breathing slow and of a snoring character, and the patient lies in a comatose condition from which he can not be roused.

Aconitum, in premonitory symptoms; violent headache above the eyes, especially when stooping or coughing.

Belladonna, if there are signs of congestion of the head and chest. A dose every hour.

Nux vomica, for persons addicted to intemperate habits, or if resulting from an overloaded stomach. A dose every hour.

GENERAL DIRECTIONS. — Remove all tight garments, raise the head, place the patient in a cool and airy apartment,

2

immerse the feet in hot water, and send immediately for medical aid.

APPARENT DEATH.

TREATMENT — Apparent death from inhaling NOXIOUS GASES. If a person has become insensible from inhaling *Carbonic Acid*, *Carbonic Oxide*, *Fumes of Burning Charcoal*, *Chlorine or Sulphureted Hydrogen Gas*, expose him at once to the fresh air. Bathe the face and breast with vinegar, and let him inhale the vapor. Give strong coffee to drink; apply cold water to the head and warmth to the feet. If necessary, have recourse to Dr. Hall's method of recuscitation, as explained under "Apparent Death from Drowning." If there is congestion to the head, loss of consciousness, give *Belladonna*. A dose every twenty or thirty minutes. If the patient is excited, talks much and rapidly, give *Coffea*. Dose as Belladonna.

From COLD, always place the body in a cold room, and cover it with snow, or bathe it in ice-cold water until the limbs become soft and flexible; then place it in a dry bed, and rub briskly with flannel, at the same time try to induce artificial respiration by Dr. Hall's method, explained under the head of "Asphyxia from Drowning." As soon as there are signs of returning life, give small injections of coffee, without milk, and if the patient can swallow, give him spoonful doses of coffee to drink.

From DROWNING, place the body in a horizontal position, *face down*, with one wrist under the forehead. Now, with one hand upon the back and the other upon the abdomen, press gently for about two seconds, then turn the body well upon the side, and after a couple of seconds place it again upon the face, and repeat as before. In this way strive to induce artificial respiration by the alternate pressure upon the abdomen and rotation of the body. Meanwhile have the limbs rubbed briskly upward, and the wet articles of clothing replaced by dry, warm ones. *Antimonium tart.* is a valuable remedy in these cases. A dose every half hour.

From HANGING, CHOKING, etc., endeavor to induce artificial respiration by the same method as recommended for drowning.

APPETITE, LOSS OF.

Generally a symptom of derangement of the stomach, and of want of power or tone in the digestive organs.

Cinchona, if there appears to be no apparent derangement of the system. A dose night and morning.

Nux vomica, when loss of appetite proceeds from sedentary habits, late hours, wine, etc.; worse in the morning. A dose night and morning.

Pulsatilla, if it arises from eating rich food, pastry, etc.; worse in the evening. A dose night and morning.

GENERAL DIRECTIONS.—Drink freely of cold water, and abstain from stimulating articles of diet to create an artificial appetite. Take plenty of outdoor exercise, and observe the general directions under Indigestion.

APPETITE, VORACIOUS.

Is frequently a symptom of worm affections, dyspepsia, pregnancy, or the result of debilitating diseases.

Cinchona, when occurring during con-valescence after debilitating illness. A dose night and morning.

Cina, when connected with worm af-fections. A dose night and morning.

Nux vomica, unnatural hunger during pregnancy, or if resulting from impaired digestion. A dose night and morning. (See Indigestion, Worms.)

ASTHMA.

SYMPTOMS.—Shortness of breathing occurring in paroxysms and attended with a sensation of suffocating constric-tion of the chest, cough, and wheezing respiration.

Arsenicum.—Difficult breathing; worse at night on lying down ; oppression of the chest, and great debility ; cold sweats, etc. A dose every hour.

Ipecacuanha.—Paroxysms of suffoca-tion ; feeling of constriction, and rattling of mucus in chest. A dose every hour.

Nux vomica.—Oppression, especially in the lower part of the chest; short cough ; indigestion. A dose every two hours.

GENERAL DIRECTIONS.—When the

first symptoms of a fit appear, immerse the feet and hands in hot water, and inhale the steam ; persons liable to asthma should be very careful in their diet. (See Bad Effects of a Chill.)

BILIOUS ATTACKS—BILIOUSNESS.

SYMPTOMS.—Nausea, frequent vomiting of bile, furred tongue, bitter taste in mouth, headache, thirst, loss of appetite, bowels either constipated or relaxed, etc.

Chamomilla.—Vomiting ; thirst ; loss of appetite ; colic ; diarrhea. A dose every three hours.

Mercurius.—Nausea or vomiting of bilious matter ; bitter taste in mouth ; headache and thirst. A dose every three hours.

Nux vomica.—Pain in stomach and side ; headache ; vomiting with constipation ; furred tongue. A dose every three hours.

Pulsatilla.—Vomiting of food ; slimy or bilious diarrhea ; shivering ; bitter taste in mouth ; loss of appetite ; also, when caused by errors in diet. A dose three times a day.

7

GENERAL DIRECTIONS.—The diet for a few days after a bilious attack should be light. (See Indigestion, Vomiting, Colic, Diarrhea.)

BOILS.

SYMPTOMS. — Inflammatory, circumscribed and painful swellings immediately under the skin, terminating in the formation and discharge of matter.

Belladonna, if the boil is red and painful. A dose three times a day.

Hepar is useful to bring the boil to a head after suppuration has commenced. A dose three times a day.

Sulphur, to prevent a recurrence of boils. A dose night and morning.

GENERAL DIRECTIONS. — Apply at first a cold water dressing (a bandage wrung out of cold water applied to the part and covered with oil silk, to be renewed frequently). When matter has formed, apply a hot bread or linseed meal poultice. (See Abscess.)

BREATH, OFFENSIVE.

May be caused by a deranged stomach, abuse of mercury, decayed teeth, diseased gums, or want of cleanliness.

Carbo veg., if arising from abuse of mercury ; gums bleed readily. A dose night and morning.

Mercurius, if it arises from diseased gums or thrush. A dose night and morning.

Nux vomica, should derangement of the stomach exist ; Nux if worse in morning ;

Pulsatilla, if worse at night. A dose night and morning.

GENERAL DIRECTIONS. — Be careful with your diet, and rinse the mouth frequently with warm water. (See Indigestion, Canker in the Mouth.)

BUNIONS.

SYMPTOMS.—Inflammation on the ball of the great toe.

TREATMENT.—When the bunion becomes inflamed and painful from walking or pressure, bathe the foot in warm water, and afterward apply an Arnica lotion in the proportion of one part of Tincture of Arnica to fifteen or twenty of water. All pressure on the bunion must be avoided.

CHICKEN POX.

SYMPTOMS.—An eruption somewhat resembling small pox, but much milder in its character ; it runs its course in six or seven days ; the feverish symptoms are generally slight.

Aconitum should be used at the commencement, if there is much fever. A dose every three or four hours.

Belladonna.—Headache, sleeplessness, or if there are symptoms of congestion in the head. A dose every three or four hours.

Rhus is considered the best general remedy in this disease. A dose every three or four hours.

GENERAL DIRECTIONS.—Keep the patient cool, the room well ventilated, and let the diet be light.

CHILBLAINS.

The frequent recurrence of chilblains is an indication that the cause is constitutional, and until the tendency is removed (which can only be done under the advice of a skillful physician), the party suffering can not expect to be free from them.

CAUSE.—Great variation in the temperature.

Phosphorus is specific in many cases. A dose three times a day.

Pulsatilla, if the part swells and itches violently. A dose three times a day.

Sulphur, if the chilblains are of long standing. A dose night and morning.

GENERAL DIRECTIONS.— Rub well, until the part is quite warm, with a rag dipped in Arnica lotion (one part of Tincture of Arnica to fifteen or twenty of water). A good, old-fashioned remedy is to hold the part affected to a hot fire for as long a time as possible. If broken, dress with Spermaceti Ointment.

CHILL OR COLD, BAD EFFECTS OF A.

Difficult breathing, colic, cough, cold in the head, diarrhea, headache, hoarseness, earache, pains in the chest and limbs, sore throat, and toothache, are among the most common complaints arising from a cold or chill.

Reference has been made to most of

these under their different headings, but a few of the principal remedies against the bad effects of a chill are here inserted.

When the affections caused by a chill are *acute* and *painful* recourse should be had to Aconitum, Chamomilla, Nux, or Pulsatilla, but when there is, on the contrary, *little pain*, Dulcamara will be found suitable in the majority of cases.

Aconitum will be found suitable in toothache, faceache, or other neuralgia, with headache, congestion, violent feverish heat, etc.

Chamomilla, in headache, toothache, earache, or other excessively painful neuralgia, with agitation, violent feverish heat, moist cough, etc.

Dulcamara, in headache, affections of the sight or hearing, toothache, sore throat, gastric sufferings, moist cough, painless diarrhea, pains in the limbs, fever, etc.

Mercurius, in pains in the limbs, sore throat, affections of the eyes, toothache, earache, painful diarrhea, dysentery, etc.

Nux vomica, in fever, dry cough, dry cold in the head, dysentery, etc.

Pulsatilla, in fluent cold in the head,

moist cough, earache, fever, diarrhea, etc., and especially in the case of pregnant women.

Bad Effects of Chill—Medicines Especially Adapted.

Asthma.—Arsenicum or Ipecacuanha.

Colic.—Chamomilla, Cinchona, or Nux.

Diarrhea.—Bryonia, Dulcamara, or Mercurius.

Earache. — Chamomilla, Mercurius, or Pulsatilla.

Eyes, Inflammation of the.—Aconitum, Belladonna, or Pulsatilla.

Gastric Derangement. — Chamomilla or Dulcamara.

Headache. — Aconitum, Belladonna, or Nux.

Hearing, Difficulty of.—Belladonna, Mercurius, or Pulsatilla.

Hoarseness. — Belladonna, Chamomilla, Dulcamara, or Kali bichromicum.

Neuralgia.—Aconitum or Chamomilla.

Pains in the Limbs.—Aconitum, Bryonia, or Mercurius.

Sore Throat.—Belladonna, Chamomilla, Mercurius, or Kali bichromicum.

Toothache.—Chamomilla, Dulcamara, or Mercurius.

A dose of the appropriate medicine may be taken every four or six hours. (See Cough, Cold in the Head, Earache, etc.)

CHOLERA, ASIATIC.

SYMPTOMS.—Almost every attack of cholera is preceded by a diarrhea, which may last from a few hours to days, and which, if promptly treated, is almost always easily cured. During the prevalence of cholera, every diarrhea, however slight, should at once receive careful attention, *not so much because the patient's condition is perilous*, but to prevent its becoming so. The patient should go to bed and remain as long as the diarrhea continues, using a bed-pan when the bowels move. If the diarrhea comes on at night, it should be immediately treated, and not wait until morning, as many do, thereby losing precious time.

Aconitum.—A dose every fifteen or twenty minutes for an hour, for the premonitory diarrhea, or during the early stage of the disease ; if purging and vomiting set in with considerable violence, the mother tincture in drop-doses, or globules medicated with the tincture, should be used.

Camphora. — When the case passes gradually from choleraic diarrhea into real cholera, the patient suddenly loses strength, and looks pinched and blue, the skin becomes very cold, voice husky and deep, intense distress and anguish at the pit of the stomach. A dose every fifteen or twenty minutes.

Veratrum alb. — *Violent* and *profuse discharges of rice-water-like fluids upward and downward*, with extreme thirst for cold water in large quantities, which is vomited as soon as swallowed. A dose every fifteen or twenty minutes.

Arsenicum.—Rapid failure of strength , great anguish and burning pain in the stomach and bowels ; great thirst for cold water, drinking but little at a time. May be given in alternation with Veratrum. A dose every fifteen or twenty minutes.

Cuprum.—Cramps or convulsions, either with or without vomiting. A dose every fifteen or twenty minutes.

Carbo veg. and *Arsenicum*, if, notwithstanding the above treatment, the case runs down into a state of collapse. A dose alternately every ten minutes.

PREVENTIVE REMEDIES.—*Cuprum* and *Veratrum alb.* alternately. Every other night a dose during the epidemic.

CHOLERA MORBUS

Comes on usually at night, in hot weather, and is characterized by an attack of vomiting and diarrhea, and deranged state of the liver, setting in with great pair. in the bowels, sickness at the stomach, and vomiting of large quantities of dark-greenish, bitter-tasting substance, frequently with cramps in the stomach and bowels, sometimes extending to the feet, hands, calves of the legs, and arms.

Ipecacuanha, when the vomiting is severe. A dose every half hour.

Colocynthis.—Vomiting of green substances, with violent colic and frequent diarrheic stools. May be given in alternation with *Ipecacuanha*. A dose every half hour.

Arsenicum. — Violent pains in the stomach, great thirst, constant nausea, diarrhea, and violent vomiting of watery, bilious, or slimy, greenish, brownish, or blackish substances. A dose every half hour till better.

Cuprum, when cramps or spasms are prominent symptoms. Dose as for *Arsenicum*.

COLD—COMMON COLD OR CATARRH.

SYMPTOMS.—Commences with shiverings, followed by slight fever, pain and heaviness in the head, sensation of the nose being stuffed, sneezing, increased secretion from the nose.

COLD IN THE HEAD (DRY).

Nux vomica.—Headache ; obstruction of the nostrils ; feeling of the head being stuffed ; aching in the limbs. A dose four times a day.

COLD IN THE HEAD (FLUENT).

Arsenicum, if the discharge is thin and acrid ; nausea and prostration of strength. A dose four times a day.

Mercurius.—Frequent sneezing ; discharge of mucus from the nose ; soreness of the nose and upper lip ; headache. A dose four times a day.

Pulsatilla.—Loss of taste and smell ; secretion yellowish, greenish, thick, or offensive. A dose four times a day.

CHRONIC CATARRH.

Kali bichromicum.—Chronic catarrh, with hoarseness ; tough, stringy sputa ; chronic, inflamed, or ulcerated sore throat ; cough, etc.

Sulphur.—Chronic catarrh, with free discharge.

GENERAL DIRECTIONS. — See under "Cold on the Chest." (See Influenza.)

COLD ON THE CHEST—BRONCHITIS.

SYMPTOMS.—Fever, cough at first dry, followed by scanty expectoration, which afterward becomes more profuse ; sometimes attended with pain in the chest and hoarseness.

Bryonia. — Dry and violent cough ; shooting pains in the side ; pains in the head ; vomiting. A dose every three or four hours.

Chamomilla. — Dry cough, or with scanty expectoration, caused by tickling in the windpipe and chest ; worse at night. A dose every three or four hours

Mercurius.—Dry and shaking cough ; hoarseness ; stuffiness of the head ; perspiration accompanying the cough. Dose as for Bryonia.

Phosphorus.—Dry cough, from tickling in the throat, or with pains in the chest, and accompanied with hoarseness or loss of voice. A dose three times a day.

Pulsatilla.—Loose cough ; rattling of mucus ; worse on lying down. Dose as for Bryonia.

Antimonium tart. in the second stage, when there is much wheezing, sickness, being induced by great accumulation of mucus, with paroxysms of cough, etc. Dose as for Bryonia.

Kali bichromicum, especially in chronic cases, with accumulation of tenacious, stringy mucus difficult to expectorate. A dose three times a day.

Diseases and their Treatment.

GENERAL DIRECTIONS. — During a cold in the head or chest, put the feet into warm water on going to bed, and eat little food. Use, as a preventive, the shower-bath every morning, or sponge the body daily with cold water. (See Cough, Influenza.)

COLIC—GRIPES—BELLYACHE.

SYMPTOMS.—Severe pain in the abdomen occurring in paroxysms, sometimes attended with nausea, vomiting, constipation, or diarrhea ; little or no fever ; the pain is relieved by pressure.

Colic—Medicines Especially Adapted.

Bilious Colic.—Chamomilla, Colocynthis, or Nux.

Chill, Colic from a.—Chamomilla, Nux, or Cinchona.

Flatulent Colic.—Chamomilla, Colocynthis, Cinchona, Nux, or Pulsatilla.

Spasmodic Colic.—Belladonna, Colocynthis, or Nux.

Colic with Diarrhea.—(See Diarrhea with Colic.

Congestion.

If Colic arises from a fit of anger or passion.—(See Emotions of the Mind.)

Chamomilla.—Tearing, drawing pains, with restlessness and tossing; flatulence. A dose every hour.

Cinchona.—Distention of the abdomen; spasmodic and constrictive pains. Dose as Chamomilla.

Colocynthis.—Violent pains, compared to stabbing, cutting, or pinching; with diarrhea. Dose as Chamomilla.

Nux vomica.—Obstinate constipation; gripings and flatulence; sensation of a band round the stomach. Dose as Chamomilla.

Pulsatilla. — Diarrhea; shiverings; aggravation on sitting or lying. Dose as Chamomilla.

GENERAL DIRECTIONS.—Foment the abdomen with hot water, or apply a hot-bran poultice or warm flannel. Let the diet be light, and let all that is partaken of be warm. (See Indigestion.)

CONGESTION, OR DETERMINATION OF BLOOD TO THE HEAD.

SYMPTOMS.—The head feels full and heavy; headache mostly over the eyes.

increased by stooping, coughing, etc.; the beating of the arteries of the head is felt by the patient; giddiness.

Aconitum, Belladonna, in most cases will prove sufficient. A dose alternately every one to four hours.

Nux vomica, should congestion to the head arise from indigestion, sedentary habits, constipation, or spirituous liquors. A dose every two to four hours.

GENERAL DIRECTIONS.—As preventives, take daily exercise, abstain from heating and stimulating drinks, and make a free use of cold water both internally and externally. (See Congestive Headache.)

CONSTIPATION.

Simple costiveness does not indicate a diseased condition, but may arise from eating much animal food, perspiration, or a sedentary life.

Bryonia, especially in summer; in constipation from disordered stomach, with headache. A dose night and morning.

Mercurius.—Unpleasant taste in the

mouth; sick headache and bilious symptoms. A dose night and morning.

Nux vomica.—Headache; giddiness; ineffectual straining, or hard, knotty stools, with much straining. A dose night and morning.

Sulphur, in many cases of chronic constipation; especially in those subject to piles. A dose night and morning.

GENERAL DIRECTIONS.—Drinking a glass of cold water before breakfast, and two hours after every meal, moderate exercise, abstinence from stimulating food and drinks, will be found valuable auxiliaries in the treatment. (See Indigestion.)

CORNS

Mostly arise from unequal pressure and often from constitutional causes. They are in general a protection of nature against undue friction upon some exposed part of the foot. This friction and pressure must therefore at once be removed before any relief can be obtained and every means adopted to restore the skin to its natural condition.

TREATMENT.—Bathe the feet in warm water, pare the corn carefully until it is even with the surrounding skin, then apply a lotion of six drops of Tincture of Arnica to a tablespoonful of water, by means of a piece of lint or linen, or when going to bed wrap the part round with a small strip of linen soaked in the above lotion, and keep it on through the night. Repeat this for several nights in succession, rubbing in a little sweet oil, or applying a little sweet oil by means of cotton during the day. When they are constitutional, the following internal treatment will frequently be of service:

Bryonia, Rhus, if the corns are very troublesome during wet weather, or the pains are of a shooting character. A dose alternately every four or six hours.

Calcarea carb., Sulphur, should be taken to eradicate a tendency to corns. A dose occasionally.

COUGH

Arises from an irritation of the air passages themselves, or from sympathy with some other organ, as the stomach, liver, etc.

COUGH, DRY.

Belladonna.—Spasmodic cough, with or without sore throat; headache on coughing; worse at night. A dose every two or three hours.

Bryonia.—Shootings in side or pains in chest; expectoration difficult. A dose every two or three hours.

Nux vomica.—Sensation of mucus in throat which is difficult to detach; pains in stomach or side on coughing. A dose every two or three hours.

COUGH, LOOSE, WITH EXPECTORATION.

Dulcamara, especially after a chill; loose cough and easy expectoration. A dose every three hours.

Pulsatilla, easy expectoration or rattling of mucus in chest; loss of voice. A dose every three or four hours.

Sulphur, in obstinate cases, with copious expectoration. A dose three times a day.

Diseases and their Treatment.

COUGH, WITH HOARSENESS.

Mercurius.—Hoarseness ; sore throat ; dry and shaking cough. A dose three times a day.

Phosphorus.—Hoarseness ; cough with pain in chest ; loss of voice. A dose three times a day.

Carbo vegetabilis.—Cough on taking the least cold ; obstinate hoarseness, or loss of voice.

Kali bichromicum.—Cough, with ·very tough expectoration, preceded by great wheezing, accompanied by difficult breathing, and followed by dizziness.

COUGH, WITH SORE THROAT.

Belladonna.—(See Cough, dry ; Sore Throat, etc.)

Mercurius.—Dry and shaking cough. (See Sore Throat.)

COUGH, STOMACH.

Bryonia, if the cough arises after eating or drinking, with vomiting of food. A dose three times a day.

Nux vomica.—A bruised sensation in

the stomach and side, and pains in these regions on coughing. A dose three times a day.

GENERAL DIRECTIONS.—The frequent inhalation of steam is very serviceable in dry, spasmodic coughs; persons subject to cough should, as a preventive, sponge the chest daily with cold water, using brisk friction with a rough towel afterward. (See Bronchitis.)

CRAMP IN THE LEGS.

SYMPTOMS.—Sudden contraction of the muscles of the calf of the leg, frequently the result of indigestion.

Nux vomica, if it arises from or is connected with indigestion. A dose two or three times a day.

Rhus, if the attacks occur by day as well as by night. A dose two or three times a day.

Veratrum, especially if with a feeling of being unable to bear the warmth of the bed. A dose two or three times a day.

GENERAL DIRECTIONS.—Press the foot firmly against some hard substance, as the wall, floor, or bedstead. Sometimes immediate relief is obtained by rubbing the limb downward with Spirits of Camphor.

CROUP.

SYMPTOMS.—Commences as a common cold, followed in a day or two with difficult breathing, and with the peculiar characteristics of the disease, *a ringing metallic cough*, noisy crowing inspiration, and obstructed respiration; frequently fatal in a few hours.

Aconitum. — Burning heat; thirst; short, dry cough; hurried breathing. A dose every one or two hours.

Hepar.—Rattling of mucus; cough loose; without much fever; feeling of suffocation from phlegm. A dose every two hours.

Spongia.—Hollow, dry, ringing cough; noisy respiration; fits of choking. A dose every two hours.

Aconitum and *Spongia* may be given in alternation, and may be administered every fifteen minutes in very acute cases.

GENERAL DIRECTIONS.—Put the child into a warm bath immediately.

DEAFNESS, CATARRHAL.

Difficulty of hearing frequently arises from or is the result of a cold or chill.

Mercurius will generally afford relief. A dose every four hours.

GENERAL DIRECTIONS.—Keep the part warm and well covered with flannel. If there is great dryness and want of wax, a little glycerine on cotton wool may be carefully inserted.

DIARRHEA.

SYMPTOMS.—Looseness of the bowels, sometimes attended with colic and vomiting; often a salutary effort of nature to remove noxious matters from the system, and, if slight, need not be interfered with.

DIARRHEA, BILIOUS.

Chamomilla.—Thirst; bilious vomiting; colic; evacuations like beaten up eggs; loss of appetite. A dose three times a day.

Mercurius. — Foul tongue; nausea; bilious eructations; gripings; straining

before or at an evacuation. A dose
three times a day.

DIARRHEA, FROM A CHILL.

Bryonia. — Especially when arising
from cold drinks. A dose three times
a day.

Dulcamara.—In most cases of diarrhea from a chill, even if colic is present. A dose three times a day.

Chamomilla, *Mercurius.*—(See Bilious
Diarrhea.)

Pulsatilla. — Liquid, slimy, whitish
evacuations, or if arising from indigestion, or errors of diet. A dose three
times a day.

DIARRHEA, PAINLESS.

Cinchona is sufficient in most cases,
especially when attended with great
weakness. A dose every six hours.

DIARRHEA, VIOLENT, WITH VOMITING.
(*English Cholera.*)

Arsenicum.—Burning pains in stomach ; great thirst ; vomiting ; weakness ;
symptoms worse after eating. A dose
every hour.

Diarrhea in Children.

Veratrum.—Coldness of the body; cramps; severe colic; vomiting. A dose every hour.

Phosphorus. — Chronic diarrhea, **or** diarrhea of a painless character, especially in old persons, or consumptive individuals. A dose three or four times **a** day.

If Diarrhea is the result of grief, fright, or a fit of anger or passion, see "Emotions of the Mind."

GENERAL DIRECTIONS. — The diet must be confined to farinaceous articles, and all food must be taken cold. (See Bad Effects of a Chill.)

DIARRHEA IN CHILDREN.

Chamomilla is one of the best remedies if the purging occurs during teething, or where the action of the skin has been suddenly checked by cold, or when the food disagrees in any way, and the motions are green, offensive, or slimy, and when there is severe pain in the bowels, causing the child to scream, to be restless, and to draw its legs upward toward the belly.

This remedy may be given singly, **or**

alternately with Ipecacuanha or Mercurius ; if relief is not soon obtained, the Mercurius is particularly indicated, if the stools are slimy and green, or if they are pap-like, or streaked with blood.

Cinchona, in simple, summer diarrhea is very efficacious. A dose three or four times a day.

Mercurius. — Green or clay-colored stools. A dose three or four times a day.

Veratrum.—Choleraic diarrhea, with watery discharges ; accompanied with severe vomiting, debility, etc. A dose every hour.

DIPHTHERIA.

SYMPTOMS. — Diphtheria, although common to children, attacks persons of any age, usually commencing with severe cold, with fever and sore throat. The illness progresses rapidly, and is marked by prostration out of proportion to the length of time that the patient has been sick. In mild cases the throat is simply red and swollen, like quinsy or scarlet fever, or ulcerated like the old-fashioned ulcerated sore throat. These cases generally yield readily to the remedies prescribed for sore throat.

The real characteristic of diphtheria, however, is a false membrane that covers the tonsils and soft palate ; *this membrane forms rapidly in patches*, which soon spread and coalesce, thus covering, in a short time, the whole throat, and extending down the larynx. The patient then finds difficulty in breathing, and is almost totally devoid of the power of swallowing.

The fetid breath is a constant symptom of an alarming character.

The *sudden prostration, the characteristic membrane, and the peculiar odor of the breath* will distinguish *diphtheria from common sore throat, from scarlet fever, from quinsy, and from the so-called ulcerated sore throat.*

TREATMENT.—*Belladonna* and *Mercurius iodatus*, in alternation, in first stages, or milder form of diphtheria, with sore pains, scraping sensation of thickness ; burning or stinging in the throat ; contraction and spasmodic constriction of the fauces ; violent stitches in the throat and tonsils, especially when swallowing ; swelling of the gums and tongue. A dose every one or two hours, alternately.

Kali bichromicum and *Mercurius iodatus*, in alternation, are generally the most successful remedies in diphtheria in the more severe form, or more advanced stages of the disease, and should be given in the first triturations, one or two grain doses, from one to two hours apart.

These remedies should be continued, in alternation, for at least twelve hours, lengthening the time between the remedies as the disease abates.

Aconitum, if the febrile symptoms run high. A dose occasionally, in connection with the other remedies.

The external application of the saltwater bandage (covered with flannel) should not be omitted during treatment ; the patient, if old enough, should gargle frequently, with lukewarm salt-water, or with a solution of Kali chloricum (Chlorate of Potassa) one part, to sixteen parts of water.

DIET. — Rich broths, wine whey,

brandy and water, etc., should be administered in proportion to the failing strength of the patient. The *nourishing diet* should be adopted *from the very beginning*.

This terrible disease requires the prompt attention of a reliable homœopathic physician.

DYSENTERY.

SYMPTOMS. — Dry skin and tongue; thirst and other symptoms of fever; frequent painful desire to stool, with great straining (*tenesmus*), with discharge of blood or blood and mucus; constipation.

Aconitum.—If febrile symptoms are well marked, the early use of this remedy often arrests the disease; at its onset, it should be administered several times; at short intervals, the mother tincture or first dilution should be used, or globules medicated with mother tincture.

Mercurius sub-corrosivus. — Bloody evacuations, with pain and extremely severe straining.

Colocynthis, after or in alternation with Mercurius when the colicky pains occur periodically, are very severe, and the discharges are mixed with green matter or lumps.

Ipecacuanha. — Autumnal dysentery, with nausea, severe straining, and colic; the evacuations first slimy, afterward bloody.

Administration in severe cases, a dose every twenty or thirty minutes; in mild, every two to four hours.

GENERAL DIRECTIONS.—Let the diet be very light. Apply a warm bran poultice to the abdomen if there is much pain.

EARACHE.

Generally the result of cold, and frequently accompanied with toothache.

Chamomilla. — Lancinating pains; dryness of the ears, especially when caused by a cold. A dose every two hours.

Mercurius.—Shooting pains extending to teeth and cheeks; discharge of wax. A dose every two hours.

Pulsatilla.—Pains with redness, swelling, and heat of the ear; with humming in the ear. A dose every two hours.

Ears, Inflammation of the.

General Directions. — Put a few drops of glycerine or sweet oil on cotton, and place in the ear ; keep the part warm. (See Bad Effects of a Chill.)

EARS, HUMMING IN THE,

Frequently arises from congestion of blood to the head, from catching cold, etc.

Belladonna, if arising from congestion to the head.   A dose three times a day.

Nux vomica, if worse in the morning. A dose three times a day.

Pulsatilla, if worse in the evening. A dose three times a day.

General Directions.—As this troublesome symptom is mostly connected with some general complaint, as cold, congestion, or indigestion, these ailments should be referred to.   (See Congestion to the Head, Earache, Indigestion.)

EARS, INFLAMMATION OF THE.

Symptoms.—Great pain in the ears, followed by swelling and redness both inside and out.

Aconitum, if there is much fever. A dose every four or six hours.

Pulsatilla is the principal remedy in this painful ailment. A dose every four or six hours.

GENERAL DIRECTIONS. — Diet light, and, if the pain is very severe, apply heated flannels or a hot bran poultice to the part affected. Persons subject to inflammation of the ears should avoid draughts of air, and should protect the internal ear from all irritation of noise or wind.

EMOTIONS OF THE MIND.

Disorders frequently arise from violent passions and emotions of the mind, as from fright, grief, or passion. These ailments require special remedies adapted to the cause from which they spring.

BAD EFFECTS OF FRIGHT.

Aconitum, if fainting, convulsions, or palpitation result from fright. A dose every hour or two, according to circumstances.

Erysipelas.

Ignatia, if diarrhea is the result of a fright. A dose three times a day.

Ignatia, if diarrhea or headache arises from grief. A dose three times a day.

Chamomilla is the most suitable remedy if colic, diarrhea, dyspepsia, headache, jaundice, or spasms are the result of a fit of anger or passion. A dose every three or four hours, according to circumstances.

GENERAL DIRECTIONS. — In many cases a tendency to strong mental emotions may be very much corrected by hygienic rules, cold bathing, exercise, etc., and individuals subject to them should do all in their power to brace and strengthen the system.

ERYSIPELAS.

SYMPTOMS. — Inflammation of the skin, with fever, and shooting and burning pains ; the part is hot, swollen, and of a crimson or purplish color, which disappears on pressure ; tense and painful ; numerous *blisters* or *vesicles* are sometimes present. Erysipelas of the head is a dangerous disease.

Aconitum.—Fever ; hot burning skin ; great thirst. A dose every four hours.

Belladonna.—Burning heat, redness, and swelling of the part ; thirst ; headache ; restlessness. A dose every four hours.

Rhus, especially in vesicular erysipelas. A dose three times a day.

GENERAL DIRECTIONS.—Flour dusted over the part is often very soothing to the patient. Be careful with the diet.

EYES, INFLAMMATION OF THE.

SYMPTOMS.—Heat, pain, and redness of the eyes, intolerance of light, headache, and fever.

Aconitum at the commencement of the attack, when the feverish symptoms are severe. A dose night and morning.

Belladonna.—Redness of the whites of the eyes ; inability to bear the light ;

pains round the eyes or in the head.   **A** dose night and morning.

Mercurius, in slight cases when there is not much fever, or when Belladonna does not seem to afford relief.   A dose night and morning.

Pulsatilla.—Worse in the open air ; secretion of mucus ; agglutination.   A dose night and morning.

GENERAL DIRECTIONS.—Keep the eye shaded, and bathe it frequently with warm milk and water.   (See Bad Effects of a Chill.)

EYES, WATERY,

Frequently arises from a general **weak**ness of the organ, and this form only **is** here treated of.

Sulphur will often be found of **benefit**. A dose every night.

GENERAL DIRECTIONS. — Bathe **the** eyes frequently in cold water, and attend to the diet.   The general **health** having much to do with weak **eyes, it** would be advisable to follow the general directions under the article on **Indiges**tion.

Diseases and their Treatment.

EYELIDS, INFLAMMATION OF THE.

SYMPTOMS.—Redness, swelling, and soreness of the lids, external and internal.

Belladonna.—Swelling and redness of the lids, with constant agglutination. A dose night and morning.

Hepar.—Redness of the lids, with nightly agglutination. A dose night and morning.

Pulsatilla.—Redness of the lids; secretion of mucus; nocturnal agglutination. A dose night and morning.

GENERAL DIRECTIONS.—Bathe the part affected with warm milk and water.

EYELID, STY ON THE.

SYMPTOMS.—A small boil situated on the eyelid.

Pulsatilla.—At the commencement, before the formation of matter. A dose night and morning.

Hepar.—When suppuration has commenced. A dose night and morning.

GENERAL DIRECTIONS.—Bathe the eyelid with warm water, and when matter has formed, apply a hot poultice.

FACE-ACHE. (TIC-DOULOUREUX.) (*Neuralgia.*)

SYMPTOMS. — An affection of the nerves of the face, usually of an acute, lancinating character; often commencing at the ear, or under the eye, and frequently an obscure and complicated disease.

Aconitum.—Redness and heat of the face; great restlessness and irritation. A dose every two hours.

Arsenicum.—Pains, very severe, with prostration of strength; worse after a meal; relieved by external heat. A dose every two hours.

Belladonna.—When the pain is most violent under the eye; darting pains in cheek bones and jaws; pains extending into the ball of the eye. A dose every two hours.

Cinchona.—In periodical attacks; aggravated by the slightest touch. A dose every two hours.

GENERAL DIRECTIONS.—Attend to diet; sponge the face well every morning with cold water, as a preventive, and as an auxiliary in the treatment.

(See Toothache, Bad Effects of a Chill.)

FACE, SWOLLEN,

Generally arises from a chill, toothache, or gum-boil.

Chamomilla.—Swelling hard ; face hot and red.   A dose night and morning.

Mercurius.—If the glands are swollen and painful, and there is a flow of saliva from the mouth.   A dose night and morning.

GENERAL DIRECTIONS.—Foment the face with hot water.

FAINTING.

GENERAL DIRECTIONS.—Remove all tight articles of clothing ; lay the patient on the floor ; dash cold water over the face, and let her smell *Spirits of Camphor.*   The room must be well ventilated.

If fainting is the result of a fright, see Emotions of the Mind.

FATIGUE, BODILY.

Great bodily fatigue mostly produces

Fatigue.

a sensation of general lassitude, and feeling as of contusion in the muscles and joints, sometimes accompanied with sleeplessness and complete prostration.

Arnica, internally, is the most suitable remedy against the bad effects of great bodily fatigue, walking, rowing, etc. A dose every four or six hours.

Aconitum should be taken against the bad effects of *overheating* from bodily exercise in summer time. A dose occasionally.

GENERAL DIRECTIONS.—Mix a tablespoonful of Tincture of Arnica in a small wash-hand basin full of tepid water, and bathe the hands and feet in it. Care should be taken if food is required, and, if extremely exhausted, to have a light meal, and to eat sparingly. The moderate use of a stimulant may sometimes be beneficial.

FATIGUE, MENTAL.

SYMPTOMS. — Over-study or watching frequently produces confusion of thought, headache, drowsiness, or sleeplessness, with general lassitude **and** weariness.

Nux vomica is the principal remedy, and will generally afford relief. A dose three times a day.

Coffea, if there is much nervous excitement and sleeplessness. A dose occasionally.

GENERAL DIRECTIONS.—Perfect rest should be given to the mind after too great a strain upon its powers; cold bathing should be resorted to, and every endeavor made to invigorate the system. Years of nervous debility and misery frequently result from an over-taxation of the mental powers.

FEVER, SIMPLE.

SYMPTOMS. — Weariness, shivering, pains in the limbs, followed by burning heat, thirst, quick pulse, loss of appetite, etc.

Aconitum will generally be found sufficient in simple feverish symptoms. A dose two or three times a day.

GENERAL DIRECTIONS. — The diet should be light, consisting merely of barley water, thin gruel, or arrowroot.

Fevers, Acute.

FEVERS, ACUTE.

Under this head are inserted a few general directions for the guidance of the patient until medical advice is obtained, as, in all cases of sudden and acute inflammatory attacks, the symptoms are of too severe a character for the treatment of any but the skillful practitioner.

SYMPTOMS.—The first symptoms of an acute attack of fever are the same as those recorded under Simple Fever, which are followed or accompanied by those symptoms which relate to the specific character of the fever to which they belong: as pains in the limbs in Rheumatic Fever; bilious symptoms in Gastric Fever; great prostration of strength in Typhus Fever; various eruptions in Eruptive Fevers, etc. In all cases of acute fever, the treatment is the same at the commencement.

Aconitum should be given at once when the feverish symptoms run high. A dose every hour or two.

Belladonna, if the head is affected;

delirium. A dose every hour or two, or in alternation with Aconitum.

GENERAL DIRECTIONS.—Put the patient to bed, keep the room cool **and airy,** give cold water to drink, barley water or thin gruel for nourishment, and send for a homœopathic physician.

FEVER AND AGUE.
(*Intermittent Fever.*)

SYMPTOMS.—The cold stage is preceded by languor, yawning, drowsy headache, numbness of toes and fingers, and blue nails ; then coldness of the extremities, gradually increasing, until the patient begins to shake and tremble, his teeth to chatter. During this time the pulse is weak and oppressed ; thirst variable; the cold stage lasts from twenty minutes to three or four hours, and varies much in intensity. The hot stage has all the symptoms of an acute inflammatory attack ; hot, dry skin ; full, quick pulse ; congestion of the head ; sometimes delirium.

Aconitum, if the febrile symptoms are very severe. A dose every half-hour until better.

Fever and Ague.

Cinchona.—Nausea and thirst before the fever; voracious appetite; headache; palpitation of the heart; thirst between the cold and hot stages, or after the hot stage; no thirst during the heat; great debility; yellow complexion. A dose every two or three hours.

Arsenicum.—*Great debility;* disposition to vomit, or violent pains in the stomach; imperfect development of chilliness and heat, or both; drinking very often, but little at a time; pains in the limbs, or all over the body, with anxiety and restlessness; oppression in the chest; nausea; bitter taste in the mouth. A dose every two or three hours.

Ipecacuanha and *Pulsatilla.*—Much shivering, with little heat, or the contrary; little or no thirst; disordered stomach; nausea, and other gastric symptoms. A dose, alternately, every two or three hours.

Nux vomica.—Bowels constipated; the paroxysms generally coming on every day, or every other day, generally in the afternoon, evening, or night, with aching pain in the forehead ; vertigo ; nausea, and bitter taste ; spasms of the stomach, and great weakness.

FLATULENCY.

SYMPTOMS.—Wind in the stomach or bowels. This symptom of indigestion frequently arises from flatulent food, drinking coffee or tea in excess, or from rich or unwholesome articles of diet.

Cinchona, when arising from flatulent food. A dose night and morning.

Nux vomica, especially when the symptoms come on after drinking. A dose night and morning.

Pulsatilla, if caused by eating rich or greasy food. A dose night and morning.

GENERAL DIRECTIONS.—Be cautious with diet, and avoid those articles of food which experience teaches you tend to promote the complaint. (See Indigestion.)

GIDDINESS

May arise from indigestion, debility, or congestion of the brain.

Belladonna.—Giddiness arising from

congestion of blood to the head. A dose night and morning.

Cinchona, if giddiness arise from debility. A dose night and morning.

Nux vomica.—Giddiness in the open air; after a meal; worse on stooping, or in the morning. A dose night and morning.

Pulsatilla.—Worse in the evening; relieved in the open air. A dose night and morning.

GENERAL DIRECTIONS.—A free use of cold water, both in drinking and sponging, and plenty of exercise in the open air, are recommended as preventives to ordinary giddiness.

GLANDS, SWOLLEN OR INFLAMED.

Often caused by a cold or chill, and this form only is here treated of. Chronic enlargement of the glands denotes deep-seated constitutional disease, which requires a lengthened course of treatment.

Belladonna, when there is bright redness of the part, and inflammation. A dose night and morning.

Mercurius, when the glands are hard.

red, hot, and painful to the touch. A dose night and morning.

GENERAL DIRECTIONS.—Keep the part warm and well covered with flannel.

GOUT

Generally affects the joints of the great toe, which become red, hot, and swollen, with burning pains.

Bryonia.—Red and shining swelling, with shooting pains ; worse on movement. A dose night and morning.

Pulsatilla, when the pains pass rapidly from one joint to another. A dose night and morning.

GENERAL DIRECTIONS. — Diet very low, and foment the part with warm water, or wrap it in cotton wool. (See Rheumatism.)

GUM-BOIL

May be caused from a decayed tooth, a cold, or from some derangement of the digestive organs.

Belladonna, if there is much redness and inflammation. A dose night and morning.

Hepar, when suppuration has commenced. A dose night and morning.

Mercurius, when the boil is hard and painful. A dose night and morning.

GENERAL DIRECTIONS.—Place a warm fig on the boil in the mouth, keep the face tied up with a handkerchief, frequently bathe the cheek, and rinse out the mouth with warm water.

GUMS, BLEEDING OF THE.

Sometimes a symptom of derangement of the stomach, but frequently arising from abuse of mercury.

Carbo veg., if it arises from the abuse of mercury. A dose night and morning.

Mercurius, in most cases (except when arising from the abuse of this mineral), especially when the gums are spongy, swollen and painful. A dose night and morning.

GENERAL DIRECTIONS.—Avoid medicated dentifrices, and clean the teeth frequently with a soft brush. (See Canker in the Mouth.

HEADACHE.

Headache may arise from various

causes, as derangement of the digestive organs, catarrh, congestion of the brain, nervous debility, etc. It is frequently only a symptom of disease, which must be cured before relief is obtained.

HEADACHE, BILIOUS AND GASTRIC.

(*Sick Headache.*)

Bryonia.—Aching pains in the forehead, or one-sided headache; constipation; nausea or vomiting. A dose three times a day.

Ipecacuanha.—Nausea; vomiting of food or bilious matters. A dose three times a day.

Nux vomica.—Nausea and sour vomiting; headache especially over the eyes; giddiness; constipation. A dose three times a day.

Pulsatilla.—Nausea or vomiting of food; semilateral headache. A dose three times a day.

HEADACHE, CATARRHAL.

Belladonna.—Great fullness in the head, especially over the eyes; excessive sensibility to the least noise. A dose three times a day.

Mercurius.—Fullness of the head; discharge from the nose, etc. A dose three times a day.

Nux vomica.—Headache and heaviness in forehead with obstruction of nose. A dose three times a day.

HEADACHE, CONGESTIVE.

Belladonna.—(See Catarrhal Headache.)

Bryonia.—Headache with feeling of compression in the head; constipation. A dose three times a day.

Nux vomica.—Headache especially over the eyes; constipation; giddiness; feeling of sleepiness. A dose three times a day.

HEADACHE, NERVOUS.

Coffea, if brought on by excitement. A dose three times a day.

Ignatia, if caused by grief; momentary relief on movement. A dose three times a day.

Nux vomica.—Worse in the morning; excited by mental emotions or fatigue;

and increased in the open air or after eating. A dose three times a day.

Pulsatilla.—Worse in the evening; relieved in the open air; increased indoors or by lying down. A dose three times a day.

HEADACHE, PERIODICAL.

Sulphur in most cases will prove efficacious. A dose three times a day.

HEADACHE, RHEUMATIC.

Chamomilla.—Tearing pains on one side of the head, extending to the jaw. A dose three times a day,

Bryonia.—Shooting pains, worse on movement or during changeable weather. A dose three times a day.

If Headache is the result of grief or passion.—(See Emotions of the Mind.)

GENERAL DIRECTIONS.—Attend to diet, and in catarrhal headache, bathe the forehead with warm water; in nervous, lie down quietly in a dark room; use cold bathing as a preventive. (See Bad Effects of a Chill.)

HEART, PALPITATION OF THE,

Often arises from mental emotions, nervousness, indigestion, or debility; thcugh frequently produced by disease of the heart, or some other organ of the body.

Cinchona, if arising from debility. A dose night and morning.

Nux vomica.—In robust persons; if worse after food, with symptoms of indigestion. A dose night and morning.

Pulsatilla.—In nervous persons, especially females, when produced by the slightest cause. A dose night and morning.

If Palpitation arise from fright.—(See Emotions of the Mind.)

GENERAL DIRECTIONS.—Avoid all excitement, abstain from coffee, strong tea, and all indigestible articles of food. Running and quick walking are injurious, especially up-hill, and soon after a meal.

HEART-BURN.

SYMPTOMS.—A painful, burning sensation of the stomach, extending up into the throat; arising from indigestion.

Diseases and their Treatment.

Nux vomica, especially if the result of sedentary habits or abuse of spirituous liquors. A dose three times a day.

Sulphur will in most cases relieve violent heart-burn, or may be given after Nux. A dose three times a day.

GENERAL DIRECTIONS.—A tumbler of cold water will often relieve the oppressive, burning pain. Those who suffer from heart-burn and waterbrash should adhere closely to the general directions laid down under the article on Indigestion.

HICCOUGH—HICCUP

May be frequently relieved by holding the breath for a few seconds, or by drinking cold water or sugar and water. Should these means not succeed, take a dose of Nux.

HOARSENESS

Generally accompanies, or is the result of, a cold.

Belladonna. — Hoarseness, with inflammation of the throat, or with cold in the head, amounting to loss of voice. A dose night and morning.

Hooping Cough.

Carbo veg.—Obstinate chronic hoarseness; worse in damp weather; after talking; and in the evening. A dose night and morning.

Dulcamara.—Hoarseness arising from exposure to damp or wet. A dose three times a day.

Hepar, in chronic cases, with or without a dry cough. A dose night and morning.

Mercurius, if connected with a cold in the head, sore throat, or cough. A dose night and morning.

Phosphorus.—Dryness and soreness of the throat and chest, especially in chronic cases. A dose two or three times a day.

Pulsatilla, with loose cough; pains in chest; thick discharge from nose. A dose night and morning.

GENERAL DIRECTIONS. — Wash the neck and throat frequently with cold water. (See Cough, Bad Effects of a Chill, Loss of Voice.)

HOOPING COUGH.

SYMPTOMS.—Is divided into three stages; first, the symptoms of a cold;

second, the cough is distinguished by its convulsive and suffocative character, occurring in paroxysms, and attended with a peculiar hooping sound; third, the cough becomes loose, and the hoop ceases.

Belladonna.—Dry, hard cough, with marked cerebral disturbance; sore throat. A dose three times a day, according to circumstances.

Ipecacuanha.—Danger of suffocation; bluish face; accumulation of phlegm on chest. A dose three times a day.

Drosera,* when the peculiar hooping cough is fully developed; vomiting of food; no fever. A dose three times a day.

Cuprum. — Paroxysms of hooping cough, causing convulsions, rigidity, and almost a suspension of the breath; followed by vomiting and extreme prostration.

Pulsatilla, in the third stage, when the cough is loose. A dose two or three times a day.

* Drosera being only recommended for hooping cough in this manual, is not included in tl.e list of remedies. It can be procured separately.

Hysterics—Indigestion.

GENERAL DIRECTIONS.—The diet in the first stage should be light, and in the second, nutritious. Change of air will be found of great service in this complaint.

HYSTERICS.

GENERAL DIRECTIONS.—Place the patient in a recumbent position on a large bed, or on the floor ; remove all tight articles of clothing which impede the circulation ; sprinkle the face with cold water ; admit plenty of fresh air, and let the patient smell Camphor, or give a dose of *Ignatia*. Persons subject to hysterical attacks should avoid all tight articles of clothing, and should follow the instructions laid down under the article Indigestion.

INDIGESTION

May be caused by overloading the stomach, eating too quickly, unwholesome food, a sudden emotion, a chill, etc.

Indigestion frequently arises from an infraction of dietetic rules, and from partaking of food which does not agree with the stomach, in which case it may merely assume the form of a *casual attack;* but, from continued neglect, the digestive powers may become impaired, and chronic indigestion or dyspepsia, with its multitudinous attendant sufferings, be the result.

A *casual attack* of indigestion resulting from an abuse of certain foods requires special remedies, according to the nature or the character of the cause which has produced it, as in

Derangement of the Stomach by Eating or Drinking.

Pulsatilla, if it arises from fat substances, pork, etc.

Nux, if it arises from coffee.

Arsenicum or *Pulsatilla*, if it arises from fruits or ices.

Pulsatilla, if it arises from pastry.

Nux, if it arises from wine, etc.

Rhus, if it arises from shell fish, muscles, etc.

If Nettlerash should be the result of partaking of unwholesome food—(See Nettlerash.)

Indigestion.

Derangement of the Stomach by Moral Causes.

Chamomilla, if it arises from anger or passion.

Aconitum, if it arises from fright.

Ignatia, if it arises from grief.

Cinchona or *Nux.*—Indigestion arising from debility.

Bryonia or *Nux.*—Indigestion arising from sedentary habits.

Indigestion arising from cold or chill. (See Bad Effects of a Chill.)

A dose of the appropriate medicine may be taken every four or six hours, according to circumstances.

Symptoms. — Heart-burn, flatulence, nausea, or sickness, pains in the bowels, palpitation, headache, etc.; one, many, or all of these symptoms may be present, and for the treatment of them individually, refer to their several headings. A recapitulation of the most prominent symptoms resulting from indigestion, with the medicines which will be found most serviceable in each, is here subjoined:

Diseases and their Treatment.

Bilious Symptoms require Chamomilla, Mercurius, or Nux.

Colic.—Nux, Pulsatilla, or Colocynthis.

Constipation.—Bryonia or Nux.

Diarrhea.—Pulsatilla.

Flatulence.—Cinchona, Nux, or Pulsatilla.

Headache.—Bryonia, Nux, or Pulsatilla.

Heart-burn.—Nux or Sulphur.

Nausea or *Vomiting.* — Ipecacuanha, Nux, or Pulsatilla.

Nightmare.—Nux or Pulsatilla.

Palpitation.—Nux or Pulsatilla.

Waterbrash. — Calcarea carb., Carbo veg., or Nux.

Bryonia.—Indigestion in individuals having a tendency to membraneous inflammations, rheumatism, etc., or when it manifests itself in summer; constipation. A dose night and morning.

Cinchona.—Indigestion arising from debility, caused by loss of blood, purging, etc. A dose night and morning.

Hepar is almost a specific (with occasionally a dose of Sulphur) in chronic or long-standing dyspepsia. A dose occasionally.

Ipecacuanha.—Indigestion, with nausea

or vomiting as a prominent symptom.
A dose three times a day.

Nux vomica.—One of the best medicines for indigestion, and especially adapted for individuals of a lively, energetic, sanguine temperament, with a predisposition to constipation or piles.
A dose night and morning.

Pulsatilla.—Like Nux vomica, but especially suitable to females or persons of a mild disposition, with tendency to a relaxed state of the system, diarrhea, etc. A dose night and morning.

Sulphur.—In most cases of chronic dyspepsia or indigestion in individuals of a nervous and irritable temperament, with tendency to piles. A dose occasionally.

GENERAL DIRECTIONS. — The best rules to avoid indigestion are: to rise early, drink a glass of cold water at once, and then sponge yourself from head to foot with cold water, rubbing the skin thoroughly dry afterward, and taking exercise in the open air if possible; but if not, in the house until thoroughly warm. Wear sufficient clothing; take three meals a day, a hearty

breakfast, a substantial dinner, and sup-
per light ; let your diet be plain and
wholesome ; avoid a variety of dishes,
all high-seasoned articles and condiments, and any thing you find to dis-
agree with you ; eat slowly, masticate
thoroughly, drink sparingly, and in general take water with your dinner ; for
breakfast and tea, weak tea or cocoa ; a
glass of water two hours after a meal
will assist digestion ; exert neither mind
nor body for some time after a meal ;
take a walk daily, the best time is between breakfast and dinner ; refrain
from stimulants and aperients ; retire to
bed early, and cultivate a cheerful, con-
tented disposition. "A merry heart
doeth good like a medicine." (See Bad
Effects of a Chill.)

INFANTS, DISEASES OF.

Acidity of the Stomach.

SYMPTOMS.—Known by looseness of
the bowels, the evacuations often of a
greenish color ; great restlessness.

Chamomilla will, in most cases, be
sufficient. A dose three or four times
a day.

Asthma of Millar—Colds.

GENERAL DIRECTIONS.—Give the child sufficient exercise, and diminish the quantity of food.

Asthma of Millar. (*Spasmodic.*)

SYMPTOMS.—Distinguished from Croup by coming on suddenly (the child frequently waking up with it), by the transient character of the attack, and by the absence of fever.

Chamomilla. — Shortness of breathing, agitation, and crying; distension of the stomach. A dose every hour.

Ipecacuanha.—Danger of suffocation, with bluish face. A dose every hour.

*Sambucus.**—When the attack comes on during sleep; dry cough and crying. A dose every hour.

GENERAL DIRECTIONS. — Apply a sponge dipped in hot water to the throat. (See Croup.)

Colds.

Imprudent exposure to cold and ir-

---

* Sambucus is not included in the list of remedies, being only recommended in this disease. It can be procured separately.

regularity of clothing are the chief causes of this ailment.

Chamomilla.—Obstruction of the nose, with running of water from nose ; cough. A dose three times a day.

Nux vomica.—Dry obstruction of the nose. A dose three times a day.

GENERAL DIRECTIONS.—If the skin is rough, use a little cold cream or Glycerine.

Colic or Crying.

SYMPTOMS.—Griping ; the infant draws its legs up to its stomach.

Chamomilla.—In colic, when the face is red, or if diarrhea is present. A dose every three or four hours.

Pulsatilla, when the colic is accompanied with vomiting, nausea, or diarrhea. A dose every three or four hours.

Colocynthis.—Colic of griping, flatulent character. A dose every three or four hours.

Nux vomica.—Colic, with constipation, accompanied with sudden fits of crying.

GENERAL DIRECTIONS.—Give the child a warm bath, and keep it well covered.

Constipation

Frequently results from errors in diet.

Bryonia, when constipation occurs during summer time, or when the motions are of a large size. A dose night and morning.

Nux vomica, when there is much straining, with hard, knotty stools. A dose night and morning.

GENERAL DIRECTIONS.—Use friction with the hand over the abdomen.

Convulsions

Mostly occur during dentition, from excitement of the nervous system, or errors in diet.

Belladonna.—Starting when asleep ; rigidity of the limbs ; drowsiness ; pupils dilated. A dose every four hours.

Chamomilla.—Convulsive jerking of the limbs ; constant movement of the head ; redness of one cheek. A dose every four hours.

If convulsions or spasms arise from fright or passion—(See Emotions of the Mind.)

Diseases and their Treatment.

GENERAL DIRECTIONS.—Put the child into a warm bath as soon as possible.

Diarrhea—Bowel Complaint.

If during dentition, and not excessive, or injuring the child's health, need not be checked ; it often results from errors in diet.

Arsenicum, if there is much emaciation, weakness, and pallor. A dose three or four times a day.

Chamomilla.—Bilious diarrhea ; colic ; restlessness. A dose three or four times a day.

Ipecacuanha, if accompanied with vomiting. A dose three or four times a day.

GENERAL DIRECTIONS.—Alter the diet and diminish the quantity. Mix a little isinglass with the child's food.

Cholera Infantum and Summer Complaint.

Cholera Infantum is sudden in its attacks. It appears in summer from extreme heat, and in autumn from hot days and cool nights. Vomiting is a precursor and a companion of the intestinal evacuations. The discharges from the bowels of a *colorless* and *inodorous fluid,* or mucus, and looking like beaten eggs, or sometimes green.

SUMMER COMPLAINT.—There is but little difference between this disease and cholera infantum except that it is *not so sudden in its invasion,* and is more insidious in its course; but cholera infantum, if not quickly checked, will degenerate into summer complaint.

Camphora and *Veratrum* alternately every hour when the child is suddenly taken with vomiting and purging. If not better in eight hours,

Ipecacuanha and *Chamomilla* in alternation. A dose every hour.

Colocynthis. — Green vomiting, with violent colic. A dose every hour.

Arsenicum.—Violent vomiting and *di arrhea,* with severe pains in the abdo men; *thirst, restlessness, sudden prostra tion.* A dose every hour till better.

Aconitum may be given in alternation with any other remedy whenever fever is present; also for great restlessness and dry heat of the body.

Diseases and their Treatment.

Excoriation of the Skin.

Often the result of a want of cleanliness.

Chamomilla is generally sufficient to remove the affection. A dose night and morning.

GENERAL DIRECTIONS. — Wash frequently in warm water, and dry the child well with a soft towel.

Heat Spots—Infant Rash.

SYMPTOMS.—An eruption frequently caused by too much clothing, or errors in diet, and generally very slight.

Aconitum, should the feverish symptoms run high. A dose three times a day.

Rhus, if the eruptions should be extensive. A dose three times a day.

GENERAL DIRECTIONS.—Sponging the skin frequently with warm water, and a proper attention to ventilation, are generally sufficient to remove the rash.

Jaundice

Frequently arises from cold, or is the result of an abuse of purgative medicine.

Mercurius will generally be found sufficient to remove it. A dose every three or four hours.

GENERAL DIRECTIONS. — Attend to diet; keep the child moderately warm. Cleanliness and warm clothing are likewise necessary.

Sleeplessness—Restlessness.

Often a symptom of general derangement, teething, etc.

Belladonna, if the child cries for hours without closing the eyes, or sleeps for a few minutes, waking up with starts. A dose at bed-time.

Chamomilla, when colic and great restlessness are present. A dose at bed-time.

Coffea. — Sleeplessness from excitement; redness of face. In most cases of sleeplessness this remedy will be sufficient. A dose at bed-time.

GENERAL DIRECTIONS.—A warm bath will frequently be found soothing.

Teething, Fever during.

The fever which is sometimes present during teething is generally slight and of a remittent character.

Diseases and their Treatment.

Aconitum.—Heat; burning of skin; thirst; sleeplessness. A dose occasionally.

Chamomilla.—Tossing; restlessness; redness of cheeks; cough. A dose occasionally.

GENERAL DIRECTIONS. — The child should be kept on a light diet, and in a quiet and airy room.

Teething, Tardy.

SYMPTOMS.—In difficult teething the face is hot and red, and the gums at the spot where the tooth wants to pierce are hard and swollen.

Calcarea carb. is serviceable when the teeth are slow in coming. A dose night and morning.

GENERAL DIRECTIONS.—Attention to the infant's diet, and guarding against undue exposure, will be of essential service.

Thrush—Aphthæ.

SYMPTOMS. — Small ulcers on the tongue, sometimes extending through the whole of the intestinal canal.

Inflammation.

Mercurius should be given in almost all cases. A dose night and morning.

Sulphur should follow Mercurius if necessary. A dose night and morning.

GENERAL DIRECTIONS. — Use the greatest cleanliness ; wash out the mouth frequently with warm water; attend to ventilation, regularity of the bowels, and taking the child into the open air as often as the weather will allow.

INFLAMMATION, ACUTE.
(*Of Internal Organs.*)

Most of the diseases which come under this heading require prompt medical assistance ; the remedies here mentioned under each particular inflammation are only intended to be used until a physician arrives.

BLADDER, INFLAMMATION OF THE.

Recognized by a burning pain in the region of the bladder, the external parts being swollen, hot, tense, and painful to the touch, the urine is hot and red, and the emission of it is either difficult and painful or impossible ; fever.

Aconitum should be taken until the

physician arrives.   A dose every one or two hours.

BOWELS, INFLAMMATION OF THE.

Recognized by violent stitching pains in the inflamed part, which are permanent, the abdomen is bloated, hot, and painful to the touch, quick, small, wiry pulse, obstinate constipation, and violent thirst.

Aconitum, Belladonna, should be taken until the physician arrives.   A dose alternately every one or two hours.

BRAIN, INFLAMMATION OF THE.

Recognized by a violent pain in the head, or by a mere pressing, dull sensation, fever, and signs of sanguineous congestion to the head, distention of the veins of the head and throat, etc.; coma or constant delirium.

Aconitum, Belladonna, should be taken until the physician arrives.   A dose every hour or two in alternation.

BRONCHIA OR AIR TUBES, INFLAMMATION OF THE.

Recognized by a constant and violent

irritation, tickling cough, and hoarse voice, attended with fever. (See **Bronchitis.**)

KIDNEYS, INFLAMMATION OF THE.

Recognized by severe, pressing, pungent pain in the region of the kidneys, with shootings from that region to the bladder; difficulty of urinating; the urine is red and hot; there is mostly vomiting, colic, and straining, and the pains are increased by motion, or by lying on the back or side affected.

Aconitum should be taken until the physician arrives. A dose every hour.

LIVER, INFLAMMATION OF THE.

Recognized by a burning and stitching pain in the right side, which extends to the shoulder and breast-bone, and sometimes even to the right foot. The pain and short dry cough attendant upon the disease are increased by inspiration, and it is impossible to lie on the right side. *This is when the inflammation affects the outer side of the liver.*

Or recognized by a deep-seated, painful pressure, rather than of pain in the region of the liver, accompanied by yellow color of the eyes and face, sometimes almost complete jaundice, bitter taste, vomiting, and high-colored urine. Fever accompanies these symptoms. The pains are increased by lying on the left side, but are alleviated by lying on the right. *This is when the inflammation affects the inner side or substance of the liver.*

Aconitum, while the fever is high. A dose every two hours.

Bryonia, Mercurius, when the fever is not very high, or when it has been subdued by *Aconitum.* A dose alternately every two hours.

LUNGS, INFLAMMATION OF THE.

Recognized by stitches or pain in one part of the chest, increased by inspiration, and hindering deep breathing, oppression of the chest, and a continuous dry cough, which is excited by speaking, and by every deep breath. The cough is afterward attended with expectoration, of a serous or mucous character, and in the highest degrees of the inflammation, pure blood may be expectorated.

Inflammation.

All the signs of inflammatory fever **are** generally present.

Aconitum, either alone or in alternation with other remedies where inflammatory symptoms run high. A dose every one or two hours.

Bryonia.—Labored, short, catching, and rapid breathing; stinging, shooting, or burning pains in the side, aggravated by inspiration; cough dry and painful. A dose every two or three hours.

Phosphorus.—Pains in the chest of a severe, sticking character, increased by coughing; breathing short; cough dry. A dose every two or three hours.

Antimonium tart.—Greatly oppressed breathing; cough with much rattling of mucus; nausea; profuse expectoration; violent throbbing of the heart, and a feeling of suffocation. A dose every one or two hours.

PLEURA, INFLAMMATION OF THE.

Recognized by painful stitches in **the** side when moving or drawing breath, attended with inflammatory symptoms. (See Pleurisy.) There is also a kind of pleurisy which is not accompanied with inflammatory symptoms. (See **False Pleurisy.**)

STOMACH, INFLAMMATION OF THE.

Recognized by a constant, burning, stitching pain in the region of the stomach, increased by inspiration, pressure of food, with tension and swelling, and frequently pulsation. There is great anxiety, restlessness, with retching and vomiting of whatever is taken ; also, violent thirst, great prostration, coldness of the limbs, and sometimes fainting or convulsions.

Aconitum, *Bryonia*, should be taken until the physician arrives. A dose alternately every two hours.

GENERAL DIRECTIONS.—Until the arrival of the physician, and while taking the medicines recommended as suitable, the patient should observe the same rules as under Fever. Water, thin gruel, or barley-water may be given to drink, the room should be airy and cool, and not too light, and every thing that may excite the patient should be carefully removed.

INFLUENZA.

SYMPTOMS.—Commences with shiverings, pains in limbs, headache, followed by obstruction of the nose, frequent sneezing, discharge from the nostrils, sore throat, hoarseness, cough, loss of appetite, great debility, etc.

Arsenicum.—Great weakness ; cough ; nausea ; fluent and acrid discharge from nose.   A dose three times a day.

Mercurius.—Sore throat ; fluent discharge from nose ; dry cough ; swelled glands.   A dose three times a day.

GENERAL DIRECTIONS.—Keeping in bed for a day or two, according to the severity of the attack, is desirable, and in other respects treat as for cold in the head.   (See Cold in the Head.)

INJURIES.

Black or Bloodshot Eye.

TREATMENT.—Bathe with a lotion of ten drops of Tincture of Arnica to a large wineglassful of water.

Diseases and their Treatment.

Bruises, Contusions, etc.

TREATMENT.—Bathe the injured part frequently by means of a rag or piece of lint dipped in a lotion composed of one part of Tincture of Arnica to twenty of water, and take one or other of the following medicines :

Pulsatilla, if the muscles are chiefly affected. A dose three times a day.

Rhus, when the joints or tendons have suffered. A dose three times a day.

GENERAL DIRECTIONS.—If the skin is broken, the lotion should be applied of only one-half the strength recommended above ; and the part affected should always be kept at perfect rest.

Burns—Scalds.

TREATMENT.—Puncture the blisters that may have arisen, and cover the whole affected part with thick raw cotton, and keep it on till the pain has left; or a Urtica urens lotion—twenty drops of Tincture of Arnica to half a pint of water—will also be found most efficacious, covering the part afterward with a thick layer of soft cotton wool, so as to exclude the air. Change the dressing as seldom as possible, the cure of burns depending so much upon the exclusion of air from the wounds.

Aconitum should be taken if there is much fever. A dose every three hours.

Hepar, if suppuration ensues. A dose night and morning.

Chapped Hands or Lips.

TREATMENT.—Rub the part well with Arnica Cerate or Glycerine, and if the hands are affected, wear kid gloves. If there is a predisposition, and the skin cracks very readily, take

Mercurius, if the lips are chiefly affected, or whenever the chaps are deep and bleeding. A dose two or three times a day.

Hepar, when the hands alone are chapped. A dose two or three times a day.

Sulphur in obstinate or long-continued cases. A dose once or twice a day.

Diseases and their Treatment.

Cuts—Wounds.

TREATMENT.—Cleanse the part thoroughly with a soft sponge dipped in cold water, as soon as the bleeding ceases, which is generally the case after the application of cold water, apply a bandage of lint, or linen moistened with a lotion of tincture of Arnica (twenty drops to a quarter pint of water) may be used in the same way, but in general Calendula is to be preferred in the treatment of lacerated wounds. Keep the injured part at perfect rest, and enjoin a low diet. If the cut is slight, unite the edges together with strips of Arnica or Calendula plaster.

Aconitum should be given if the patient is very feverish. A dose every four hours.

Cinchona, if faintness arises from loss of blood. A dose every hour.

Sprains or Strains.

TREATMENT.—Apply a bandage kept constantly moist with an Arnicated lotion (one part of the tincture of Arnica to twenty of water). The part affected must be kept perfectly at rest.

Arnica (internally) should be taken while using the Arnica lotion externally, or when the parts affected appear black. A dose three times a day.

ITCH.

Symptoms.—The real itch appears in pointed vesicles filled with a transparent serous fluid mostly about the wrists, between the fingers, and around the joints. The itching increases in the evening, especially in the warmth of the bed. It does not appear on the face.

Sulphur is generally regarded as the specific remedy. A dose two or three times a day.

Mercurius iod., if Sulphur does not cure promptly. A dose two or three times a day.

General Directions.—Perfect cleanliness, bathing and washing daily is essentially important. Sponging the parts with a weak solution of Carbolic acid and water is very beneficial.

Diseases and their Treatment.

JAUNDICE.

SYMPTOMS.—Loss of appetite, bitter taste in the mouth, furred tongue, skin of a yellow color, constipation or diarrhea, evacuations light in color, depression of spirits.

Mercurius is the principal remedy, and will generally afford relief. A dose every three or four hours.

Cinchona, if the disease should not yield to Mercurius, or if that drug has been taken to excess. A dose every three or four hours.

Chamomilla.—Jaundice in passionate or fretful patients, especially children. A dose every three or four hours.

Nux vomica.—Jaundice with constipation, sensitiveness in the region of the liver, and for patients of sedentary or intemperate habits. A dose every three or four hours.

If Jaundice arises from a fit of anger or passion.—(See Emotions of the Mind.)

GENERAL DIRECTIONS.—Keep quiet, observe a light diet, and drink only water or toast and water. Take an occasional warm bath.

LUMBAGO.

SYMPTOMS. — Rheumatism affecting the muscles of the back.

Bryonia, when the pains are worse during motion. A dose night and morning.

Nux vomica, when the back feels as if bruised ; aggravated by motion ; constipation. A dose night and morning.

Rhus.—Worse when at rest, or just beginning to move. A dose night and morning.

GENERAL DIRECTIONS.—Use friction every morning, and wear a flannel bandage round the part. Take care of your diet, as Lumbago is often connected with indigestion. (See Rheumatism.)

MEASLES.

SYMPTOMS.—At first resemble those of a cold in the head ; on the fourth day small red points appear in crescentic clusters, first on the face and then on other parts of the body. The eruption disappears in four or five days.

Aconitum, when the feverish symptoms are intense. A dose three or four times a day.

Pulsatilla is the specific for Measles, and may be employed as soon as the feverish symptoms are diminished, or in alternation with Aconite. A dose three or four times a day.

Bryonia.—Imperfectly developed or suppressed eruption ; stitching pains in the chest ; difficult breathing ; cough, etc. A dose every three or four hours.

Sulphur.—To complete the cure, if, after the Acon. and Puls., chronic cough, etc., should remain. A dose night and morning.

GENERAL DIRECTIONS.—Diet light ; room well ventilated, but not cold.

MENSTRUATION, DISORDERS OF.

Slight disorders of the monthly period are here alone treated of. Long standing, complicated, or habitual irregularities, should have competent medical advice. A non-observance of the general principles of hygiene will be found a fruitful source of much of the suffering attendant upon these functions.

Menstruation, too soon.

Colic, Menstrual,

Is frequently caused by a chill from dampness of the feet, errors in the mode of living, and an imprudent use of drugs.

Chamomilla, *Pulsatilla*, are the best remedies for Colic during the monthly period.

GENERAL DIRECTIONS. — See under "Painful Menstruation." (See Colic, Painful Menstruation.)

Menstruation, too soon.

Frequently produced by mental emotions, excesses of various kinds, great bodily exertion and over-fatigue.

Calcarea carb., when there is a tendency toward increasing shorter intervals, the flow also increasing in proportion. A dose three times a day.

Nux vomica, especially if the flow lasts too long, and is profuse ; cramps. A dose three times a day.

GENERAL DIRECTIONS.—A hard bed, plenty of fresh air, salt-water baths, salt-water sponging, and every thing that can invigorate and strengthen the system, should be resorted to.

Diseases and their Treatment.

Menstruation, Painful,

Arises from cold, deficient exercise, insalubrity of air, a sudden emotion, etc.

Chamomilla, if there are colicky pains, with bearing-down feelings and tenderness of the abdomen. A dose every six hours.

Nux vomica, if the forcing pains predominate. A dose every six hours.

Pulsatilla, if occurring in individuals of a mild and timid temperament. A dose every six hours.

GENERAL DIRECTIONS. — A careful diet, frequent walking, muscular exercise, all sorts of amusements, and absence of all violent and unpleasant emotions are indispensable requisites to a cure.

Menstruation, too Profuse.

The causes of this irregularity are both mental and physical, and are similar to those which are productive of painful or too frequent menstruation.

Cinchona, if attended with great weakness. A dose every three or four hours.

Ipecacuanha, if the discharge is very

profuse, and amounts to flooding. **A** dose every quarter of an hour to **an** hour.

Nux vomica, when the discharge is excessive and lasts too long. A dose every three or four hours.

GENERAL DIRECTIONS.—The patient should remain perfectly quiet, and all drinks should be given cold. If flooding sets in, medical aid must be procured.

Menstruation, Retarded or Suppressed.

This condition frequently arises from a sudden emotion, a violent disappointment, a chill or cold (especially arising from damp feet), bad air, fatigue, etc.

Aconitum, when there is headache, giddiness, or congestion, especially in robust young women. A dose every two or three hours.

Pulsatilla is the principal remedy, especially when the suppression is the result of a chill. A dose every two or three hours.

GENERAL DIRECTIONS.—A warm hip or foot-bath may be used, and when the acute symptoms are removed, active exercise in the open air should be resorted to, care being taken to clothe the body in a manner suitable to the season, and to avoid thin soles to the shoes and getting the feet damp.

MILK CRUST.

SYMPTOMS.—An eruption mostly confined to infants while nursing, consisting of small, white pustules in clusters on a red ground, appearing first on the face, and sometimes spreading over the whole body. The pustules burst, and form yellow scabs, and are attended with considerable irritation.

Aconitum, when there is great fever and restlessness. A dose two or three times a day.

Rhus is specific in many cases, and is particularly indicated when the itching is very troublesome. A dose two or three times a day.

Sulphur should be given to aid the cure, or if *Rhus* has not produced a favorable change. A dose night and morning.

GENERAL DIRECTIONS.—The diet of both mother and child must be most carefully attended to. Observe great cleanliness, and bathe the part affected with tepid water, to allay the irritation.

MOUTH, CANKER IN THE.

SYMPTOMS.—Gums are hot, swollen, red, and tender; become spongy and shrink from the teeth; frequently ulcers form on them, and the smell from the mouth is offensive.

Carbo veg., if arising from abuse of Mercury, or if the gums bleed much. A dose night and morning.

Mercurius will be found sufficient in ordinary cases. A dose night and morning.

GENERAL DIRECTIONS. — Attend to your diet, keep the mouth clean, and avoid medicated dentifrices.

MUMPS.

SYMPTOMS.—Swelling of the glands behind the ears and under the jaws, attended with fever, headache, etc.

Belladonna, if the swelling is very red, or if there are symptoms of the brain being affected. A dose every four hours.

Mercurius will suffice in all ordinary cases. A dose three times a day.

GENERAL DIRECTIONS.—Keep flannel to the part ; avoid all exposure to cold, and live sparingly.

NERVOUS EXCITEMENT.

CAUSES.—The nerves of some persons are naturally weak and delicate, but many bring themselves into this distressing condition by a neglect of the general laws of health, thereby entailing upon themselves the hundred distressing symptoms this complaint often assumes.

Chamomilla, when there is great irritability of disposition. A dose night and morning.

Coffea, when there is great excitability, with sleeplessness and restlessness. A dose three or four times a day.

GENERAL DIRECTIONS.—All persons who suffer from this complaint should avoid late hours, crowded assemblies, all kinds of mental excitement, novel reading, and the like ; let them eschew coffee, strong tea, and stimulants, and live, if possible, in the country ; rise early in the morning, and retire to rest before ten at night; sponge the body daily with cold water ; take brisk exercise in the open air ; and let the diet be plain, wholesome, and nourishing. (For Nervous Debility, see Weakness.)

NETTLE-RASH.

SYMPTOMS.—An eruption resembling that caused by the sting of nettles, and attended with itching; it seldom remains many hours in one part; frequently arises from indigestion or a cold.

Dulcamara, when it arises from a cold. A dose night and morning.

Calcarea carb., if the rash disappears in the open air; and in chronic cases. A dose night and morning.

Rhus, if it arises from unwholesome food, or from damp weather. A dose night and morning.

GENERAL DIRECTIONS.—Avoid any article of diet which seems to produce it, and use warm water only, externally, to allay the irritation. (See Bilious Attacks, Indigestion.)

NIGHTMARE.

SYMPTOMS.—A sensation of weight on the chest, felt during sleep, impeding respiration, and producing great anxiety, or accompanied with horrid dreams or fancies.

Aconitum, if attended with fever and palpitation of the heart. A dose or two before going to bed.

Nux vomica, when produced by sedentary habits, spirituous liquors, and the like. Dose as *Aconitum*.

Pulsatilla, when arising from late suppers, and rich articles of food. Dose as *Aconitum*.

GENERAL DIRECTIONS.—Late suppers and a want of power in the digestive organs being fruitful sources of this painful affection, individuals subject to it should avoid the one and try to increase the tone of the other. (See Indigestion.)

NOSE, BLEEDING FROM THE.

Sometimes a salutary effort of nature relieving headache, giddiness, etc.

Belladonna, when there are symptoms

of congestion of the brain ; flushing of the face ; fullness of the vessels of the head. A dose every three or four hours.

Rhus, if in consequence of physical exertion. A dose every three or four hours.

GENERAL DIRECTIONS. — Use cold water freely to the nose and face ; a key or some other cold substance to the back of the neck will frequently stop the bleeding.

PILES.

SYMPTOMS. — Small tumors formed from a distended condition of the veins situated at the rectum, either external or internal ; they may be *blind* (*i. e.*, not bleeding) or *bleeding ;* constipation is generally present ; they are always constitutional.

Nux vomica.—Especially when they exist in persons of sedentary habits, or who have indulged to excess in coffee or spirituous liquors. A dose three or four times a day.

Sulphur.—After *Nux*, especially when

the tumors burn and frequently protrude. A dose three or four times a day.

Nux and *Sulphur* may be given in alternation.

GENERAL DIRECTIONS. — Attend to diet, carefully avoiding stimulating food, and take a warm bath to allay the pain, or sit over a vessel of hot water.

PIMPLES.

SYMPTOMS.—The common name of a very frequent eruption, consisting of small pimples containing matter, occurring chiefly on the face, and generally the result of errors in diet. (See Boils.)

Belladonna, especially when they occur in young people. A dose night and morning.

Sulphur, in most cases, will prove beneficial, or may be given if *Belladonna* does not prove sufficient. A dose night and morning.

GENERAL DIRECTIONS.—The cause of these disfiguring little blotches must be removed before a cure can be obtained. Those who are troubled with them should abstain from spirituous liquors, take less animal food, and see that the diet is light, wholesome, and nutritious. (See Indigestion.)

PLEURISY.

SYMPTOMS. — Inflammation of the membrane lining the chest; characterized by fever, shooting pain in chest, increased by coughing or pressure; **dry cough**; shortness of breathing.

Aconitum should be given while the fever, pain, and cough are severe. A dose every three or four hours.

Bryonia, if, after the *Aconite*, sharp pains still remain in the side. A dose every three or four hours.

Sulphur, to complete the cure; if the side should still remain sensitive to the impression of the air, or to movement. A·dose night and morning.

GENERAL DIRECTIONS.—The patient should remain in bed, and the diet must consist of farinaceous articles, gruel, barley water, etc.

PREGNANCY, DISORDERS INCIDENTAL TO.

During the state of pregnancy, women are subject to certain special ailments, but they generally enjoy an immunity from the severer forms of disease.

Colic.

A very frequent trouble, which often sets in during the first months, and is frequently the result of cold or improper diet.

Chamomilla is generally successful in affording relief. A dose every three or four hours.

Nux vomica, if *Chamomilla* is not sufficient, or if the bowels are very costive. A dose every three or four hours. (See Colic.)

Constipation

Should be attended to and remedied, as much harm may arise from too great straining at stool.

Bryonia, Nux vomica, will generally be found successful in removing this condition. A dose two or three times a day.

GENERAL DIRECTIONS.—A change of diet, more vegetables and fruit, exercise, and a free use of cold water should be resorted to ; and should the bowels prove very obstinate, an injection of warm water, in which a little Castile soap has been dissolved, may be had recourse to.

Diarrhea.

This condition requires to be carefully guarded against, as having a tendency to bring on miscarriage.

Chamomilla will frequently be found of benefit, especially if there is colic. A dose every four or six hours.

Pulsatilla may follow *Chamomilla*, if that remedy has not produced the desired effect. A dose every four or six hours.

GENERAL DIRECTIONS. — The diet should be light, and should be taken in small quantities at a time ; keep the bowels warm and well covered with flannel.

Toothache

Sometimes lasts from the commencement to the end of pregnancy, and is frequently the first symptom from the presence of which that state is suspected.

Diseases and their Treatment.

Chamomilla, if the pain proceeds from a hollow tooth, or is most violent at night. A dose every three or four hours.

Nux vomica, if the pains are rendered worse by wine, coffee, or mental work. A dose every three or four hours.

Pulsatilla, if the whole side of the jaw is affected, or the pains shift about. A dose every three or four hours.

GENERAL DIRECTIONS. — The teeth should not be extracted, as the pain will not be relieved by doing so.

Varicose Veins

Result from pressure consequent upon pregnancy. After delivery, the pressure being removed, the veins regain their natural size, and the swelling disappears.

Pulsatilla is the specific in this affection. A dose three times a day.

Sulphur may be given after *Pulsatilla*. A dose night and morning.

GENERAL DIRECTIONS.—The patient should not stand too long at a time, and all tight garters and the like should be avoided. A laced stocking, giving an equal pressure all round the leg, may be used, and should be drawn on in the morning before the veins are distended.

Vomiting or Nausea.   (Morning Sickness.)

A very common symptom of pregnancy, which generally begins at the commencement, and lasts until the third or fourth month.   It sometimes, however, continues longer, or recurs periodically during the whole course of pregnancy.

Arsenicum.—Excessive vomiting, with fainting or great weakness.   A dose every three or four hours.

Ipecacuanha, if the vomiting continues very long and the patient rejects every thing she takes; or if the bowels are relaxed at the same time.   A dose every four hours.

Nux vomica, in a large number of cases, the best remedy.   A dose every four hours.

GENERAL DIRECTIONS. — The diet should be carefully regulated, and a change made in the times of eating to those hours when the stomach is less

apt to be sick. Cold food will some
times be retained when warm articles
of diet are rejected. Plenty of fresh
air and exercise are indispensable during pregnancy.

QUINSY.

SYMPTOMS.—Swelling, redness, and
inflammation of the tonsils, with difficulty of swallowing and feverish symptoms.

Aconitum at the commencement, if
the feverish symptoms are severe. A
dose every four hours.

Belladonna. — Great thirst; bright
redness of the throat; swelling of the
glands outside the throat; difficult deglutition. A dose every four hours.

Mercurius. — Shooting pains in the
throat, extending to the ears; flow of
saliva; foul taste in mouth; ulcers in
throat; shiverings. A dose every four
hours.

Mercurius iodatus is the best form of
Mercury in this disease.

Belladonna and *Mercurius* may be
given in alternation.

Rash.

GENERAL DIRECTIONS.—Relief is often afforded by the inhalation of steam.

RASH.

Purple or Scarlet Rash is, in its general symptoms, similar to Scarlet Fever, except that the general bright efflorescence of the skin is accompanied with a fine rash, which imparts to the skin a sense of granular roughness when passing the hand over it. Scarlet Fever invariably appears first on the face, next on the body, and, lastly, on the extremities; Purple or Scarlet Rash, on the contrary, may appear irregularly, or locally, or at once over the whole body.

Rose Rash is the mildest of all eruptive fevers, and is characterized by a simple blush, of a rose color, appearing in oval patches upon different parts of the skin, and sometimes extending over a considerable surface. There is no elevation on the skin, and the fever is very slight.

In both kinds of Rash the treatment may be the same.

Aconitum at the commencement, when

there is fever. A dose three times a day.

Belladonna, if the head is affected. A dose every three or four hours.

Coffea, if there is much restlessness, irritability, or nervousness. A dose every three or four hours.

GENERAL DIRECTIONS.—Attention to diet, temperature, and cleanliness will conduce much to a cure.

RED GUM.

SYMPTOMS.—An eruption, common to infants at the breast, of small, red, pimples, which make their appearance about the face, neck, and arms, frequently very slight, and yielding to simple hygienic treatment, bathing, ventilation, etc.

Aconitum may be given in most cases where there is much feverish heat and restlessness. A dose two or three times a day.

Rhus, when there is much irritation or burning itching of the skin. A dose two or three times a day.

Sulphur is often a specific, or may be used occasionally during the use of other medicines. A dose night and morning.

Rheumatism.

GENERAL TREATMENT.—Guard against the child's catching cold, and wash frequently with tepid milk and water.

RHEUMATISM

Affects especially the muscles and fibrous portions of the joints; the part affected is hot and painful, frequently red and swollen; more or less fever is always present.

Aconitum, in attacks of acute rheumatism, when feverish symptoms run high. A dose three times a day.

Bryonia.—Pains, especially in the muscles; worse on movement; with headache and bilious symptoms. A dose night and morning.

Pulsatilla.—Pains which pass rapidly from joint to joint; worse at night. A dose night and morning.

Rhus, when the pains are chiefly in the tendons; worse during repose, or when commencing to move. A dose night and morning.

Sulphur, in almost all cases of chronic, and after an attack of inflammatory rheumatism, when the pains linger about. A dose night and morning.

Diseases and their Treatment.

GENERAL DIRECTIONS.—Let the diet be low, and wrap the part in cotton wool. (See Lumbago, Sciatica, Bad Effects of a Chill.)

RINGWORM—SCALD-HEAD.

SYMPTOMS. — A pustular eruption, formed in small rings, containing yellow matter. It appears most frequently on the head, but Ringworm is found on various parts of the body. The pustules burst, discharge a little fluid, and form a scab. It is usually very tedious.

Rhus, especially when the skin is inflamed and red, and there is much itching. A dose night and morning.

Sulphur may be used after Rhus, or when the eruption dries off. A dose night and morning.

GENERAL DIRECTIONS.—Cut the hair short; wash the head night and morning in tepid bran-water, and if the scabs are thick apply a poultice. All salt meats, pickles, etc., must be avoided.

SCARLATINA.

SYMPTOMS. — An eruptive fever, attended with sore throat; the eruption comes out on the second or third day, and is of a bright-scarlet redness. This disease commences with the usual symptoms of fever, attended with sore throat; on the second or third day a scarlet eruption appears—first on the face and neck, and from thence extending over the body; about the fifth day the eruption begins to peel off, and in a week it is generally gone.

Aconitum, at the commencement, if feverish symptoms run high. A dose every two or three hours.

Belladonna is the specific in uncomplicated scarlet fever. A dose every three or four hours.

Mercurius iod.—Inflamed, swollen, or ulcerated throat, especially of a malignant character. Dose as for Belladonna, or may be given in alternation with Belladonna. (See Quinsy, Ulcerated Throat, etc.)

Sulphur, when the disease is on the decline, to complete the cure. A dose night and morning, for several days.

Belladonna should be used as a disinfectant when scarlet fever is in the neighborhood, as it generally proves a specific in preventing others from taking the infection; and even should it not do this, will greatly ameliorate the attack. A dose every morning.

GENERAL DIRECTIONS. — Diet light; room well ventilated, but not cold. If the throat is very sore, inhale steam.

SCIATICA.

SYMPTOMS.—A neuralgic affection of the sciatic nerve; the pain extends from the back of the hip to the knee or foot; it is frequently connected with indigestion.

Nux vomica, if worse in the morning; constipation and bilious symptoms. A dose three times a day.

Pulsatilla.—Worse at night, and when seated. A dose three times a day.

Rhus. — Pains, with stiffness of the muscles; worse during repose, or when commencing to move. A dose three times a day.

GENERAL DIRECTIONS. — Sponging with cold water will often be of service, both as a preventive and auxiliary in the treatment. (See Rheumatism, Indigestion.)

SEA-SICKNESS.

SYMPTOMS.—Nausea or vomiting occasioned by the motion of the vessel, often attended with great debility and exhaustion.

Nux vomica should be taken the day before going on board. A dose three times a day.

Petroleum * is often a specific in this distressing ailment. A dose every hour or two.

*Cocculus.**—Great nausea, with inability to vomit. A dose every hour or two.

GENERAL DIRECTIONS.—Be on deck as much as possible, eat dry captain's-biscuits; but, if really ill, retire to bed. A wet compress bandage round the abdomen is frequently of great service in severe cases.

SHINGLES.

SYMPTOMS.—A vesicular eruption on an inflamed base, extending about half

---

* As Cocculus and Petroleum are only recommended, in this Manual, under Sea-sickness, it has not been thought necessary to include these remedies in the case of medicines; they can easily be procured just previous to a voyage.

way round the waist, attended with itching and tingling of the skin.

Mercurius is the principal remedy for this affection. A dose every three or four hours.

Rhus, when the eruption is drying up. A dose every three or four hours.

GENERAL DIRECTIONS.—Diminish the diet, and avoid cold or damp air.

SKIN, ITCHING OR IRRITATION OF THE.

An affection which sometimes exists without any apparent eruption.

Mercurius, if the irritation is worse at night, and the skin is moist. A dose night and morning.

Sulphur is sufficient in ordinary cases. A dose night and morning.

GENERAL DIRECTIONS. — Wash the body frequently with warm water, and abstain from all indigestible food.

SLEEPLESSNESS,

Apart from disease, may arise from an overloaded stomach, over-excitement, or cold feet.

Belladonna, when there is drowsiness,

with inability to sleep. A dose at bed-time.

Coffea, when produced by over-excitement. A dose at bed-time.

Pulsatilla, if from too full a meal, or gastric derangement. A dose at bed-time.

GENERAL DIRECTIONS.—Sponging the body with cold water before getting into bed will often procure sleep. Take care that the bed-room is not too hot, take plenty of outdoor exercise, and do not study late.

SMALL-POX.

SYMPTOMS. — The premonitory are, pains in the back, and nausea, with fever; on the third day, small, hard pimples appear, first on the face, and in two or three days extend over the body. From the fifth to the eighth day these pimples become converted into pustules, containing yellow matter, and having a depression in the center; about the tenth day the pustules burst and form scabs, which, in a few days, fall off. During the time the pustules are becoming perfected, the face swells, there

is sore throat, and often difficult deglu
tition.

Aconitum, during the premonitory
stage, if the fever is severe. A dose
every three hours.

Mercurius is suitable after the appearance of the pimples, especially if there
is swelling of the face, fetid smell from
mouth, and salivation. A dose every
three or four hours.

Antimonium tart.—A prominent remedy in this disease, and should be given
as soon as Small-pox is suspected. The
spasmodic retching, nausea, and hoarse
cough, often very distressing, are relieved by it. A dose every three or
four hours.

Sulphur.- Toward the end of the disease, when the scabs have formed. A
dose three times a day.

GENERAL DIRECTIONS. — Keep the
patient in a well-ventilated apartment,
exclude all light ; to relieve the itching,
paint the pustules frequently with cream,
using a camel's-hair brush.

SORE THROAT.

SYMPTOMS.—Redness and dryness of

the throat; pain on swallowing, which sometimes extends to the ears; hoarseness, occasional loss of voice, and feverish symptoms.

Belladonna.—Pain, redness, and dryness of the throat; difficult deglutition, A dose three times a day.

Mercurius.—Shooting pains, extending to the ears; foul tongue, etc. A dose three times a day.

GENERAL DIRECTIONS.—The inhalation of steam will frequently relieve the dryness and pain in the throat. Apply a cold-water bandage round the throat, which will generally afford relief. (See Bad Effects of a Chill, Quinsy.)

Sore Throat, Ulcerated.

Belladonna, Mercurius.—(See Quinsy.)
Arsenicum may be given in putrid or gangrenous sore throat, especially when attended with great weakness. A dose every two or three hours.

Sore Throat, Relaxed, with Elongation of the Uvula.

SYMPTOMS.—Sometimes the uvula or soft palate hangs lower than usual, caused by a relaxed condition of the muscles forming it. This state is generally attended with a cough, produced by a tickling in the throat; slight inflammation and sore throat.

Nux vomica, when accompanied with derangement of the digestive organs. A dose two or three times a day.

Mercurius, if it arises from a cold, with swelling of the glands. A dose two or three times a day.

GENERAL DIRECTIONS.—Pouring cold water over the back of the neck three or four times a day is beneficial.

STIFF NECK

Generally arises from a cold or rheumatism.

Bryonia, when arising from rheumatism, or when connected with rheumatism in other joints. A dose three times a day.

Dulcamara, if the consequence of exposure to damp or wet weather. A dose three times a day.

GENERAL DIRECTIONS.—Rub the neck with oil or fat, wear a piece of flannel round it, and carefully avoid all draughts or exposure to cold.

STOMACH, SPASMS IN THE.

SYMPTOMS.—An affection of the nerves of the stomach, arising from various causes, mental emotions, indigestible food, etc., and attended with spasmodic and contractive pains in the stomach, or a sensation of constriction in that organ; frequently accompanied with nausea or vomiting, and even faintness, and may be relieved or increased by taking food.

Carbo veg.—Pains increased by pressure; worse after a meal, and when lying down. A dose every four hours.

Colocynthis.—Windy spasms or spasms mitigated by bringing up wind. A dose every four hours.

Nux vomica.—Contracting, pressing, and spasmodic pains; flatulence; nausea; constipation; worse after a meal. A dose every four hours.

GENERAL DIRECTIONS.—Endeavor to promote a healthy state of digestion, and, during the attack, if severe, take a dose of *Camphor* every quarter of an hour. (See Indigestion.)

SUN-STROKE.

Arnica.—Mix twenty drops of the *mother tincture* with half a tumblerful of water.to make a lotion ; wet a piece of linen with it, and apply it to the top of the head. Also take a dose of *Aconitum* occasionally.

TEETHING, AILMENTS DURING.

The process of teething gives rise to a variety of diseases in children, which frequently cause great suffering, and are in many cases attended with danger; most of the ailments occurring during dentition are similar to those noticed under " Diseases of Infants," and generally require the same treatment. A recapitulation of the remedies will here suffice.

Coffea, if there should be agitation or restlessness.

Nux or *Bryonia*, if there should be constipation.

Chamomilla or *Mercurius*, if there should be diarrhea.

Aconitum or *Chamomilla*, if there should be fever.

Belladonna or *Coffea*, if there should be sleeplessness.

Belladonna or *Chamomilla*, if there should be spasms.

Calcarea, if the teeth are *slow* in coming.

A dose of the appropriate medicine may be given two or three times a day, according to circumstances.

GENERAL DIRECTIONS. — Attention should be paid to the food of the infant during teething, which should be simple and unirritating in its nature, and if the child has not been weaned, the mother should observe the same care with her diet. (See Diseases of Infants.)

THROAT, " CLERGYMAN'S."

SYMPTOMS.—The name given to a chronic state of hoarseness and feebleness of voice, induced by too great a strain upon the vocal powers, as in the case of ministers, singers, lawyers, etc.

Hepar, Phosphorus, Spongia.—-One or other of these medicines will be found serviceable in this ailment. A dose night and morning.

GENERAL DIRECTIONS.—The frequent local application of cold water will be found beneficial.

TOOTHACHE

Arises from various causes, as indiges-tion, rheumatism, debility, hysteria, etc

Toothache from a Cold or Chill.—Chamo milla, Dulcamara, or Mercurius.

Toothache from a Decayed Tooth.—Bel ladonna, Mercurius, or Nux.

Toothache from Indigestion.—Nux.

Toothache, Nervous.—Belladonna, Cham omilla, or Nux.

Toothache, Rheumatic.—Chamomilla oi Mercurius.

Toothache in Children.—Chamomilla.

Belladonna.—Pains which are aggra-vated in the evening, or at night after lying down ; also in the open air, and from food ; heat and redness of the face. A dose every hour or two.

Chamomilla. — Pains occupying the whole side of the face ; swelling and red-ness of the face ; the pain seems almost insupportable, especially at night.   Dose as Belladonna.

Dulcamara, when the toothache arises from a chill, especially if diarrhea is present.   Dose as Belladonna.

Mercurius.—Pains in decayed teeth occupying the whole jaw, extending to the ears, aggravated by the warmth of the bed, or after taking any thing cold. Dose as Belladonna.

Nux vomica.—Gnawing pains in decayed teeth ; worse in the open air, or if arising from a derangement of the digestive organs.   Dose as Belladonna.

GENERAL DIRECTIONS.—Cleaning the teeth and rinsing the mouth with plenty of cold water, twice and even thrice a day, is almost imperative as a preservation from toothache.   Attention to the general health is also very necessary.

URINARY COMPLAINTS.

The treatment of these disorders should be left to the medical practitioner, but in the event of sudden emergencies arising, a few hints on those forms of disease most likely to occur are here given.

Urinating, Difficulty of, or Suppression,

May result from an abuse of ardent spirits, catching cold, suppressed piles, a fright, a fall or blow, etc.

Aconitum, in inflammatory symptoms, often in alternation with some other remedy. A dose every two or three hours.

Camphora.—Spasm at the neck of the bladder, especially if caused by Cantharides. A dose every fifteen minutes for three or four times.

Nux vomica, if the difficulty has been brought on by the abuse of spirituous liquors, or from suppressed piles. A dose every hour or two.

GENERAL DIRECTIONS.—Put the patient into a hip-bath of warm water, and apply warm flannels to the region of the bladder. Give warm mucilaginous drinks, as gum or honey and water, and send for medical aid.

Urine, Incontinence of,

Frequently arises from worms, gastric derangement, too great a degree of nervous irritability, mechanical pressure during pregnancy, etc.

Belladonna.—Spasmodic incontinence of urine, especially when occurring in nervous individuals, or when it passes off at night. A dose three times a day.

Cina, if it arises from worms. A dose three times a day.

Rhus.—Utter inability to retain the urine. A dose three times a day.

GENERAL DIRECTIONS.—When it occurs in children, the quantity of fluid which they take should be diminished, and they should be roused at regular intervals to accustom them to regular times of emission. Cold sponging of the abdomen daily will be found very efficacious.

VEINS, VARICOSE (OF THE LEGS).

SYMPTOMS.—A swollen and knotted condition of the veins of the legs, which frequently occasions great pain, and is accompanied with a sensation of weight and fatigue.

Pulsatilla will generally be found of benefit. A dose night and morning.

GENERAL DIRECTIONS. — The diet

should be light and nourishing; **too** much standing should be avoided, **and** the limb, when not taking **exercise,** should be kept in a horizontal position. An elastic stocking will also be found **of** great service.

VOICE, LOSS OF.

Mostly the result of a cold, **and gen**erally a severe state of hoarseness.

Belladonna.—(See Hoarseness.)

Mercurius, when the throat feels **rough** ; worse at night, and when **every** breath of air aggravates the case. **A** dose three times a day.

Phosphorus.—Dryness of the throat and chest ; chronic loss of voice, or if connected with a cough. A dose three times a day.

GENERAL DIRECTIONS.—A cold-water bandage will frequently afford relief. (See Bronchitis, Cough, Hoarseness.)

VOMITING OR NAUSEA.

Nausea or Vomiting may arise from many causes, as inflammation of the brain, stomach, or bowels ; from indigestion, bilious derangement, etc.

Vomiting of Blood.

Ipecacuanha.—From overloading the stomach, or with diarrhea. A dose every hour or two.

Nux vomica.—From weakness of the stomach, or bilious vomiting ; constipation. A dose every two or three hours.

Pulsatilla, when produced from eating rich or greasy food ; sour bitter vomiting ; constant nausea after eating ; shiverings. A dose every two or three hours.

Arsenicum.—Violent vomiting, with colic and diarrhea. A dose every two or three hours.

GENERAL DIRECTIONS. — While the vomiting continues take no nourishment, except cold water, barley-water, or gruel ; stimulants to check the vomiting are very injurious. Should the vomiting arise from an overloaded stomach, it may be well to assist it by copious draughts of warm water. (See Bilious Attacks, Indigestion.)

VOMITING OF BLOOD.

CAUSES.—Suppression of the menses, especially at the change of life ; diseases of heart or liver ; ulcers in stomach , violence sustained externally, etc.

SYMPTOMS.—The *warning* symptoms are : giddiness ; cold legs and arms ; wind ; sense of weight, pain, fullness or anxiety at the stomach. The *actual* ones are : discharge of dark, half-digested blood, blackened by the acids of the stomach, and mixed with food or bile ; weakness ; slow pulse ; pale or sallow countenance ; yellowish hue of eyes.

TREATMENT.—This disease is of too formidable a nature to be treated, save by a homœopathic practitioner ; but until his advice can be obtained, the following medicines may be administered :

Aconitum and *Ipecacuanha* may be taken until a physician can be obtained. A dose, alternately, every fifteen minutes to half an hour, until the vomiting ceases, afterward every two hours in alternation.

WARTS.

SYMPTOMS.—Hard, corn-like excrescences, generally appearing on the fingers.

Calcarea carb., Sulphur, Rhus.—One or other of these medicines will gen-

erally succeed in dispersing these un-
sightly formations. A dose night and
morning.

WATERBRASH.

SYMPTOMS.—The vomiting of thin,
watery, tasteless, or bitter fluid; a
symptom of indigestion.

Calcarea carb., when the waterbrash
is of an acid character, and in chronic
cases. A dose night and morning.

Carbo veg.—Waterbrash, with sour
eructations. A dose night and morning.

Nux vomica, in most cases complicated with indigestion in general. A
dose night and morning. (See Indigestion.)

WEAKNESS.

Weakness arising from disease does
not come within the scope of domestic
practice; casual attacks of weakness
and exhaustion are here alone treated.

Cinchona, if arising from corporeal
exertion, with violent perspiration. A
dose every evening.

Nux vomica, after fatigue in the open

air ; hysterial and nervous debility. A dose every evening.

Ignatia, in hysterical and nervous debility ; or from the effects of grief. A dose every evening.

GENERAL DIRECTIONS.—In general debility, but especially of nervous or hysterical character, the cold bath will be found of most essential service, and should be regularly persevered in ; regular exercise in the open air is also of the greatest importance, as tending to brace the whole system.

WHITES—LEUCORRHEA,

Results frequently from a relaxing or exciting mode of living, inactivity of the body, late hours, dissipating pleasures, stimulating diet, abuse of warm baths, mental emotions, etc.

Calcarea carb., when it occurs in females of a weakly constitution, and naturally mild disposition. A dose night and morning.

Pulsatilla, in many cases, will prove of great benefit, especially if the discharge has been occasioned by fright or chill at the time of the menses. A dose night and morning.

Sulphur, in simple cases, or, to render milder, cases wherein the discharge is corrosive. A dose night and morning.

GENERAL DIRECTIONS.—It is absolutely necessary that the patient should not be exposed to cold or damp ; should be properly clothed and fed ; should avoid warm baths, too much excitement, late hours, and hot rooms.

WHITLOW.

SYMPTOMS.—A very painful abscess at the end of the finger ; the symptoms are pain, heat, swelling, throbbing, and redness ; after a few days (unless its progress is stopped by medicine) matter is formed ; it runs its course like an ordinary boil.

Mercurius.—Before the formation of matter. A dose three times a day.

Hepar should be administered if suppuration has commenced. A dose three times a day.

GENERAL DIRECTIONS.—Soak the finger in water as hot as can be borne, and kept so by being renewed from time to time, or apply cold-water dressings; when matter has formed, use instead a hot poultice. (See Abscess.)

WORMS, THREAD.

SYMPTOMS.—May exist in the intestines without giving rise to any indication of their presence, so long as the system enjoys good health. The only certain evidence of their existence is their being voided at stool. The following symptoms, however, generally indicate their presence: emaciation, paleness of the face, frequent picking of the nose, grinding of the teeth when asleep, peevishness, inordinate appetite, gnawing sensation at the stomach, abdomen hard and swollen, evacuations irregular, great irritation at the anus.

Aconitum, if feverish symptoms are present, with great itching; colic; restlessness at night. A dose night and morning.

Mercurius may follow *Aconitum*, especially if there is diarrhea, with swelling and hardness of the abdomen. A dose night and morning.

Cina—Fever; irritability; picking at

the nose; pale face, with livid circles round the eyes; discharge of pin-worms. A dose night and morning.

Sulphur may occasionally be given in alternation with the other remedies, or will be found suitable after the fever and nervous symptoms are subdued and mitigated. A dose night and morning.

GENERAL DIRECTIONS.—Avoid unripe fruit, raw vegetables, and pastry. Cold bathing and exercise in the open air are essential, as tending to improve the general health. If the worms are very irritating, use an injection of salt and water (a teaspoonful of salt to half a pint of water), or one of vinegar and water (one tablespoonful of vinegar to four of water).

PART III.

CONCISE MATERIA MEDICA

MEDICINES AND THEIR USES,

As Recommended in this Book.

I. ACONITUM NAPELLUS.

IN inflammations and fevers, and in congestions of different organs; acting especially on the circulating system, lowering the frequency of the pulse, etc. The symptoms which indicate its use are: shiverings, followed by dry, burning heat of skin; flushed face; great thirst; pulse quick and full; headache; restlessness; foul tongue; loss of appetite. Aconite is so pre-eminently the " Homœopathic lancet," that it may be given in every case where much fever is present, as in *Catarrhal, Inflammatory,*

Aconitum Napellus.

Rheumatic, and *Simple Fevers; Bronchitis, Chicken Pox, Feverish Colds, Croup, Erysipelas, Inflammation of the Ears, Inflammation of the Eyes, Gout, Measles, Pleurisy, Quinsy, Rheumatism, Scarlatina, Small Pox, Worms;* in *Asthma of Millar, Heat Spots, Milk Crust, Red Gum,* and *Teething of Infants;* also in the feverish symptoms attendant on *Burns, Scalds, Cuts,* or *Wounds;* congestions, especially to the chest, heart, and head, particularly in plethoric persons; in *Suppressed Menses,* in plethoric young women, leading a sedentary life; in *Face-ache,* with redness and heat of the face, great restlessness and irritation; also in *Nightmare,* attended with feverish symptoms; bad effects of *Fright.*

NOTE.—The medicines recommended under the heading of each complaint and condition, are those of the greatest range and importance, and are therefore the most adapted to, and likely to meet ordinary and simple cases. It not unfrequently happens, however, that simple ailments change their character, and yet are not beyond the range of domestic practice; provision has therefore been made to meet those changes, and medicines have been in every case prescribed whose operation is so specific, whose powers have been so well tested, and whose range of action is so extensive, that they will be found quite sufficient to meet all diseases likely to come within the scope of Domestic Practice. *Aconitum* and *Belladonna* are, however, so peculiarly adapted to most diseases of an acute character that the use of them may with safety be left to the judgment of the reader. They are the chief medicines in inflammations and fevers in their various forms. Wherever feverish symptoms runs high, and are of a simple inflammatory character, *Aconitum* is required ; but if with the fever the brain is affected, and there are what may be termed "head symptoms," *Belladonna* is the medicine. *Belladonna* may also safely be given in cases where there is much inflammation, with red, hot swelling of the affected part. A dose may be administered from every four to eight hours, or the two medicines may be given in alternation.

2. ANTIMONIUM TARTARICUM.

The chief sphere of action of this medicine lies in the *mucous membranes*, the *skin*, and the *lungs*. In large doses it produces a kind of catarrhal inflammation, beginning in the lining membrane of the throat and extending to the trachea and bronchial tubes, and even extending its irritant influence on the *lungs* themselves. We therefore find that Tartar emetic is a valuable remedy in certain kinds of inflammation of these parts, and in *Catarrhal Croup*, *Bronchitis*, and *Pneumonia.* It is a most useful remedy in *Small Pox*, and, if timely used, will frequently cure without any other medicine.

3. ARSENICUM ALBUM.*

Ailments characterized by excessive debility and prostration, with oppression of chest and difficult breathing, as in *Asthma*—with a thin and acrid discharge from nose, and nausea, as in *Cold in the Head*, and *Influenza*—with burning pains in internal parts, great thirst, and emaciation, as in violent *Diarrhea*, violent *Vomiting*, *Vomiting of Pregnancy*, and *Diarrhea of Infants ;* also in *ulcerated Sore Throat* when attended with great weakness. In *Face-ache*, and in paroxysms of pain with anxiety, coldness, disposition to lie down, and sudden excessive debility. In gastric derangements arising from fruits and acids, and in diarrheas either painless or attended with burning and violent colic.

* White Arsenic.

Materia Medica.

4. BELLADONNA.

In *Inflammatory, Rheumatic,* and other *Fevers,* attended with a marked inflammatory action of the brain, delirium, startings, etc. Ailments characterized by congestion of blood to various parts —to the head, as in *Congestion to the Head, Humming in the Ears, Giddiness,* and *Bleeding from the Nose*—to the head, with headache and sleeplessness, as in *Chicken Pox*—with sensibility to the least noise, as in *Congestive Headache*—with hard, dry cough and sore throat, as in *Hooping Cough*—and to the head and chest, as in *Apoplexy*. Inflammations—with disposition to suppurate, as in *Abscess* and *Boils*—with great swelling and bright redness of the part, as in *Inflammation of the Eyelids, Swollen Glands, Gumboil, Mumps, Quinsy,* and *Sore Throat,* with inability to bear the light, pains in the head, and redness of the whites of the eyes, as in *Inflammation of the Eyes*. Inflammatory affections of the nerves, as in *Toothache* and *Face-ache*. Ailments characterized by red, hot swelling, with thirst, headache, and restlessness, as in *Erysipelas;* or with a uniform, smooth, shining, scarlet redness, as in *Scarlatina.* Ailments caused by colds, as spasmodic *Cough*, with headache on coughing, or with sore throat; *Catarrhal Headache;* and in *Hoarseness* and *Loss of Voice*, attended with inflammation of the throat. Convulsive motions and spasms—spasms of children, or *Convulsions of Infants*, with drowsiness and dilated pupils. Pinching and drawing pains in the abdomen, especially about the navel, as in *Colic;* or with paleness of face and constant crying, as in *Colic of Infants.* Also, *Sleeplessness* when there is drowsiness with inability to sleep, and *Sleeplessness of Infants.* NOTE.—See note under Aconitum.

5. BRYONIA ALBA.

Ailments characterized by rheumatic and gouty tension, drawing, tearing, and stitching mostly in the limbs, especially when moving, with red, shining swelling of the part, as in *Rheumatism*, *Gout*, and *Lumbago;* also stiffness and stitches in the joints during contact and motion, as in *Stiff Neck* and *Rheumatism*, and in *Rheumatic Headaches* worse during changeable weather. In inflammations, as of the *Lungs*, *Liver*, and *Stomach*. Ailments affecting the lungs and the muscles associated with the organs of respiration—dry and violent cough, with shooting pains or stitches in the side or chest, pains in the head, and vomiting, as in *Bronchitis* and *Pleurisy*, or with difficult expectoration, as in *Cough*. Bilious and gastric complaints, as in *Headache* with aching pains in the forehead, constipation, nausea, or vomiting; in *Stomach Cough*, when the attack arises after eating or drinking, with vomiting of food; in *Indigestion* and *Constipation* occurring especially in summer time, or resulting from sedentary habits; and in *Diarrhea* arising from cold drinks. Also in *Constipation* arising from pregnancy. For the effects of a suppression of eruptions by chills; ailments from suppression of measles and scarlet eruptions; and in *Corns*, with pressure or burning stinging, or with sore feeling when touched.

6. CALCAREA CARBONICA.

Ailments connected with scrofulous and rickety constitutions, especially when there is a predominant disposition to fluent coryza, cold, and diarrhea ; or it is particularly adapted to frail individuals being poorly fed, or also to such as have in their youth a marked disposition for growing fat and stout.

Calcarea is most beneficial in affections resulting from menstrual irregularities, as *Muscular Weakness, too frequent Menstruation, Whites*, excessive irritability of the nervous system, etc.

Chronic eruptions, *Nettle-rash, Freckles, Warts*, and *Corns*. Gastric complaints, sour vomiting, heart-burn after any kind of food, vomiting of the ingesta, and *Waterbrash*. Ailments arising from dentition, as in *Slow Teething*. More particularly adapted to chronic diseases.

7. CAMPHORA.

This remedy is invaluable in the invasive stage of *Influenza*, derangements in general, with *chilliness* and *shivering*, *Malignant Cholera*, excessive, sudden prostration of the nervous system from any cause; fainting and dizziness; cramps in the legs, arms, or abdomen; severe purging. It antidotes almost all the vegetable poisons. In consequence of its volatile properties, it should be kept separate from other homœopathic remedies.

NOTE.—The Tincture of Camphor (homœopathic) will be found useful to antidote the effects of the medicines, if required; and is also most valuable at the commencement of cold in the head, influenza, bowel attacks, cholera, etc.

Administration.—The medicated globules, or two to five drops on a lump of sugar every half hour to two hours.

8. CARBO VEGETABILIS.

Ailments arising from an abuse of mercury, as in *Offensive Breath, Bleeding of the Gums*, and *Canker in the Mouth*. Ailments arising from derangement of the digestive organs, caused by eating fat meats, pork, etc.; or in *Waterbrash*, sour eructations, raising of air or bitter eructations; also in *Spasms of the*

Stomach, with burning, aching, contractive pains.

9. CHAMOMILLA.

Hypochondriac and hysteric affections, hysterical faintings, etc., also the bad effects of anger or passion. Great irritability and sensitiveness of the whole nervous system, in *Nervous Excitement*, restlessness, with anxious moaning and tossing about. Gastric and bilious affections, with either vomiting, thirst, loss of appetite, colic, or diarrhea (the evacuations like rotten eggs), as in *Bilious Attacks*, *Bilious Diarrhea*, *Colicky Diarrhea*, *Diarrhea of Pregnancy*, *Acidity*, and *Diarrhea of Infants*. Ailments caused by a chill, *Earache*, with lancinating pains and dryness of the ears ; *Swollen face* and *Face-ache*, with hard swelling ; face hot and red, or with spasmodic twitchings of the facial muscles ; or in *Toothache* caused by a chill, or occurring during pregnancy. In *Rheumatic Headache*, and in rheumatic, drawing, tearing pains, with laming, numb feeling in the affected part ;

worse at night. Pains which **appear** intolerable, aggravated by every motion: in *Colic*, with restlessness and tossing; in *Colic of Infants*, when the face is red and diarrhea is present; also in *Menstrual Colic*. Various ailments of children and new-born infants: in *Asthma of Millar*, with shortness of breathing, agitation, and crying, distension of the stomach; in *Colds*, *Excoriation of the Skin*, *Sleeplessness*, and fever during *Teething in Infants*, with tossing and restlessness; also in *Convulsions of Infants*, with convulsive jerking of the limbs, constant movement of the head, and redness of one cheek. Affections of the bronchial tubes, with dry cough and scanty expectoration, as in *Cold on the Chest*. Aching pains in the pit of the stomach, as from a stone, with great anguish and tossing, as in *Spasms of the Stomach*.

10. CINCHONA, OR CHINA.

Ailments characterized by great debility arising from excessive loss of animal fluids, blood, and humors, **as in**

Cina—Coffea cruda.

Palpitation of the Heart, Giddiness, Indigestion, Fainting arising from loss of blood in *Cuts* or *Wounds*, and in *Weakness* after severe acute diseases. In *Dyspepsia*, bilious and gastric affections, when there is impaired *Appetite*, with great weakness of digestion, *Flatulency*, bitter taste in mouth, eructations, and heart-burn, *Flatulent Colic*, or with yellow color of the skin, *Jaundice;* also in yellow, watery mucus, or *Painless Diarrheas*, or diarrheas of undigested matter. Diseases with a periodical type, as in *Face-ache*, etc.

11. CINA.

In *Worm Affections*, with sleeplessness, dilated pupils, voracious hunger, picking of the nose, or incontinence of urine.

12. COFFEA CRUDA.

Ailments characterized by excessive nervous excitability, as in *Nervous Headache, Sleeplessness, Sleeplessness of Infants, Mental Fatigue*, and *Nervous Excitement*. Excessive painfulness of the affected part, and great irritability of the body and mind.

13. COLOCYNTHIS.

In *Flatulent Colic* and for pains in various parts of the body, which take on the character of spasm, severe pains in the stomach, followed by violent purging, swelling of the stomach from wind, attended with violent pains in the bowels and restlessness of the whole body; frothy, greenish, or yellow discharges. In *Dysentery*, when the disease is located in the small intestines; stools slimy; bloody-like scrapings, with or without tenesmus during stool.

14. CUPRUM. (Aceticum or Metallicum.)

Derangements of the nervous system, characterized by *Cramps, Convulsive Movements*, etc.; *Epilepsy*, with violent convulsions, paleness of the face, dizziness, and great debility; *St. Vitus' Dance;* in *Cholera*, with *violent cramps* in the *extremities;* nausea, with violent vomiting, with cramps in the stomach and extremities, with violent diarrhea; *Hooping Cough*, long-continued paroxysms of convulsive coughing, with vomiting of mucus; blue face and lips.

15. DULCAMARA.

Ailments arising from a cold or chill, as in *Loose Cough, Diarrhea, Nettle-rash, Stiff Neck;* and *Toothache.*

16. HEPAR SULPHURIS CALCAREA.

Suppuration of inflamed parts, favoring and promoting the suppurative process, as in *Abscess, Boils, Sty, Gum-boil,* and *Whitlow.* In *Inflammation of the Eyelids*, with nightly agglutination. Catarrhal affections, with loose cough and rattling of mucus, as in *Croup;* also in *Chronic Hoarseness.* Ill effects of mercury, *Dyspepsia*, and weakness of digestion in persons who have taken much mercury. In unhealthy skin, where even slight injuries produce suppuration and ulceration. Chapped skin and cracks of the hands and feet.

Materia Medica.

17. IGNATIA AMARA.

Bad effects of fright and silent grief. Hysteric debility, as·in *Weakness, Hysterics*, and *Fainting*. Sadness, great in-difference, and apathy; taciturnity, and in ailments of individuals of a highly nervous temperament, as in *Nervous Headache*.

18. IPECACUANHA.

Paroxysms of suffocation, as in *Asthma*, with feeling of constriction and rattling of mucus in chest; in *Asthma of Millar*, with bluish face, or in *Hooping Cough*, with bluish face and accumulation of phlegm on chest. Bilious and gastric complaints, with vomiting of food or bilious matters, and loathing of food, as in *Bilious Headache, Indigestion, Vomiting during Pregnancy*, and *Vomiting* or *Nausea;* also where there is vomiting with diarrhea, as in *Diarrhea of Infants*. Hemorrhages from various organs, as in *Profuse Menstruation* and *Vomiting of Blood*.

19. KALI BICHROMICUM.

Affections of the mucous membranes and the skin. Discharges from the nose, mouth, throat, stomach, vagina, or any of the mucous membranes, of a tough, stringy mucus, which sticks to the parts, and can be drawn out into strings; cough, with expectoration of tough, stringy mucus, which sticks to the throat, mouth, and lips; the cough choking and croupy; worse in the morning. True membraneous croup. *Chronic Hoarseness.* In *Chronic Bronchitis*, with tough, stringy expectoration and burning pain in the trachea and bronchia. *Diphtheria.* Pseudo-membraneous lesions of a diphtheritic nature, affecting the respiratory mucous surfaces, nares, superior portion of the pharynx, larynx, trachea, and bronchial tubes. Especially adapted to fat, light-haired people, and to scrofulous, catarrhal, and syphilitic diseases.

20. MERCURIUS.

There are various preparations of

Materia Medica.

Mercury used in homœopathic practice, but we refer in this manual to three.

(1.) *Mercurius solubilis,* or *vivus,*

As the action of the two are so similar that they may be used indiscriminately.

Ailments connected with the mucous membranes, the glands, and the liver. Catarrhal and inflammatory affections of the respiratory organs and the lungs, as in *Cold in the Head; Bronchitis; Cough with Hoarseness; Cough with Sore Throat; Catarrhal Headache; Hoarseness,* and *Influenza,* accompanied by one or other of the following symptoms: dry and shaking cough; perspiration accompanying the cough; hoarseness or loss of voice; fluent discharge of mucus from the nose; soreness of the nose; fullness and stuffiness of the head; frequent sneezing; headache; sore throat. Inflammatory fevers, with disposition to perspire. Swelling and inflammation of the glands, as in *Swollen Face, Swollen Glands,* and *Mumps.* In *Inflammation of the Liver;* also in gastric and bilious complaints, as in *Bil-*

ious Attacks and *Constipation,* with sick headache, thickly-coated tongue, and bitter taste in the mouth ; or in mucous and *Bilious Diarrhea, Colicky Diarrhea,* and *Dysentery,* where there is straining, with evacuations of mucus or blood ; colic ; or with clammy perspiration. In various kinds of ulcers and ulcerations, and in suppurations tending to resolve the matter or to forward the suppurative process, as in *Abscess, Gum-boil,* and *Whitlow;* also in affections of the mouth and throat, as in *Offensive Breath, Bleeding of the Gums, Thrush, Canker of the Mouth,* especially where the gums are diseased and ulcers are present ; in *Sore Throat,* with elongation of the uvula, and in *Quinsy,* with ulcers, flow of saliva, and shooting pains in the throat ; also in cases where the teeth are loose, the gums are swollen and recede, and there is much salivation (except, of course, when arising from an abuse of mercury, in which case take Carbo veg.). Ailments arising from a cold or chill, *Catarrhal Deafness;* and in pains which appear intolerable, especially at night, as in *Earache, Face-ache,* and *Toothache.*

Affections of the liver, especially where the skin assumes a dingy yellow color, as in *Jaundice*, and *Jaundice of Infants.* Diseases of the skin; itching; nightly itching, aggravated by the warmth of the bed; in vesicular eruptions, as *Shingles;* and in pustular eruptions, as *Small-pox.* In worm affections, when there is diarrhea, with straining.

(2.) *Mercurius subcorrosivus.*

Dysenteric affections, with tenesmus (straining), burning pains in the abdomen, and discharge of blood and mucus; *Cirrhosis;* scrofulous, rheumatic, and syphilitic *Ophthalmia.*

(3.) *Mercurius iodatus.*

In diseases of the glandular and lymphatic system; and is the form of Mercury that should be used in diseases of the throat, as *Quinsy* and *Diphtheria,* and in syphilitic affections.

21. NUX VOMICA.

Ailments of sanguine, choleric temperaments, and persons of hemorrhoidal dispositions. Consequences of and ailments arising from sedentary habits, mental labor, and fatigue, wine, spirits, and coffee. Derangements of the digestive functions, as in *Bilious Attacks, Offensive Breath, Colic, Constipation, Stomach Cough, Cramp in the Legs, Flatulency, Giddiness, Humming in the Ears, Bilious Headache, Palpitation of the Heart, Indigestion, Heart-burn, Waterbrash, Constipation in Infants, Sea-sickness, Relaxed Sore Throat,* with elongation of the uvula, *Spasms of the Stomach, Toothache,* and *Vomiting* or *Nausea,* accompanied by one or other of the following symptoms : headache, especially over the eyes ; furred tongue ; loss of appetite ; bitter taste in the mouth ; loathing of food ; gripings ; spasmodic contractive pains in the stomach ; giddiness ; flatulency ; heartburn ; waterbrash ; slight or obstinate constipation, or knotty stools, with much straining ; nausea or sour vomiting ; or in *Apoplexy* and *Nightmare,* when caused by an overloaded stomach. In blind and bleeding *Piles.* Affections of a catarrhal character, as in *Asthma,* with oppression in the lower part of the chest, difficulty of breathing, and short cough; in *Cold in the Head, Dry Cough, Catarrhal Headache,* and *Colds in Infants,* with obstruction of the nostrils, loss of smell, sneezing, and feeling of the head being stuffed. In *Congestion to the Head,* and *Congestive,* rheumatic, and nervous headaches, with heaviness in the head, tensive aching pain in the forehead, particularly over the eyes. Rheumatic affections, as in *Lumbago* and *Sciatica,* accompanied with constipation and bilious symptoms. Hysteric and hypochondriac affections. Hysteric debility, as in *Weakness,* and in *Indigestion* arising from debility. Ailments incidental to pregnancy, as in *Constipation, Toothache,* and *Vomiting;* and in *profuse, painful,* and *too frequent Menstruation.*

22. PHOSHORUS.

Hysteric weakness and general, sudden, and excessive weakness. In catarrhal affections, and ailments affecting the respiratory organs, the throat, windpipe, and chest; stoppage and trouble-

some dryness of the nose ; hoarseness
and roughness of the throat, acute and
chronic ; *Loss of Voice; Dry Cough*,
with stinging in the throat ; pains in
the chest ; difficulty of breathing, and
anxious respiration. In *Chronic Diarrheas*, or in diarrheas of a painless
character, especially in aged persons.
In *Chilblains* on the hands and feet.

23. PULSATILLA.

Ailments principally of females, or of
individuals of a mild, sensitive temperament, with disposition to cold in the
head, and other mucous discharges.
Derangement of the digestive functions,
and disorders from rich food, pork, pastry, and fruits, as in *Bilious Attacks, Offensive Breath, Colicky Diarrhea, Flatulency, Colic, Giddiness, Humming in the
Ears*, and in *Bilious Headache, Indigestion*, and *Nausea* or *Vomiting*, accompanied by one or other of the following
symptoms : semilateral headache ; bitter
taste in the mouth ; loss of appetite, or
hunger ; coated tongue ; eructations ;
flatulency ; nausea, or vomiting of food ;

slimy, whitish, or bilious diarrhea, and shiverings. In *Sleeplessness* from too full a meal, and in *Nightmare* arising from gastric derangement. Catarrhs, with profuse mucous discharges, as in *Cold in the Head*, with loss of taste and smell; in *Bronchitis* and *Loose Cough*, with rattling of mucus—worse when lying down; also in *Hoarseness*, with loose cough and thick discharge from the nose; and in *Hooping Cough*, when the cough is loose. Gouty and rheumatic pains which suddenly shift to other parts, or which are worse at night when seated; sometimes with swelling of the affected part, as in *Gout*, *Rheumatism*, and *Sciatica*. In *Sty on the Eyelid* before the formation of matter; and in *Inflammation of the Eyes* and *Eyelids*, with redness of the lids, secretion of mucus, and nocturnal agglutination; also when there is lachrymation in the open air. In *Inflammation of the Ears*, and in *Earache* with redness of the ear, humming in the ear, swelling, and heat. Nervous affections, as in *Nervous Headaches* and *Palpitation of the Heart* in females, when produced by the slightest cause. Affections of the skin, eruptive fevers, especially *Measles; Chilblains* with blue-red swelling, heat, and burning throbbing. In *Painful* or *Suppressed Menstruation*, and in *Menstrual Colic;* also in *Diarrhea, Toothache,* and *Vãricose Veins* during pregnancy.

24. RHUS TOXICODENDRON.

Rheumatic and gouty tension, drawing and tearing in the limbs—worse during rest, or when beginning to move —as in *Rheumatism, Lumbago,* and *Sciatica.* Lameness in all the joints, worse on rising from a seat after having been seated for some time. Stiffness of the limbs on first moving the limb after rest. Laming stiffness in the extremities when first moving a part, as in *Cramps in the Legs. Erysipelas, Nettle-rash, Scaldhead, Ringworm, Shingles, Heatspots, Milk Crust, Red Gum,* and other eruptions, especially vesicular, forming scurfs with burning itching; small burning vesicles with redness of skin on the whole body. In *Incontinence of Urine,* especially during rest, when the urine passes off involuntarily. Bad effects of a strain, dislocation, concussion, and other mechanical injuries, as in *Sprains* or *Strains*, *Bruises*, and *Bleeding from the Nose.* Affections of the tendons, membranes, and ligaments. *Warts*, and *Corns* with burning and soreness.

25. SPONGIA.

In *Croup* with hollow, dry, ringing cough ; noisy respiration ; fits of choking.

26. SULPHUR.

Affections principally in persons of a lymphatic constitution, subject to eruptions, enlarged glands, etc., or else of a bilious constitution, with disposition to hemorrhoids, to hypochondria and melancholy. Chronic diseases in general. Chronic disorders of the digestive organs, as in *Indigestion, Constipation,* and *Heart-burn;* chronic *Rheumatic* affections ; chronic and *Periodical Headaches;* also in chronic *Cough* with copious expectoration. In *Piles* and hemorrhoidal affections. Scrofulous complaints, curvature of bones, affections of

Sulphur.

the glands, eruptions and skin diseases, *Scald-head, Ringworm, Irritation of the Skin, Milk Crust, Pimples, Red Gum, Small-pox,* particularly during the suppurative stage, *Boils, Warts, Corns, Chaps,* etc.; also, *Chilblains* of long standing, or with redness, swelling, and suppuration, or with itching on warmth. Sulphur has long been known as the specific for *Itch. Cramps in the Leg* and contraction of the limbs. In *Dysentery,* with straining at stool, and evacuations of mucus and blood. Blisters in the mouth, and in *Thrush;* also in *Worm* affections. In *Varicose Veins* during pregnancy, and in *Whites* when the discharge is acrid. Ailments of persons with any constitutional taint. Sulphur exerts so great an influence over the whole system, that there are but few chronic ailments in which it is not required as well to commence the treatment as to predispose the system to the action of other medicines more especially indicated, and often in acute cases to remove effects which do not seem to yield to other remedies, as in the treatment of *Measles, Pleurisy,* etc.

27. VERATRUM ALBUM.

In *Cramps in the Legs*, with cramps and pains which do not bear the warmth of the bed ; and in *Violent Diarrhea* with severe colic, vomiting, and coldness of the body ; *Cholera Symptoms*, cold, clammy sweats, pulse slow and almost extinct, great weakness, coldness, and shivering.

With a view of rendering the uses and action of the various medicines more plain, the organs of the body which they specially affect, and the temperaments, habits, and conditions for which they are peculiarly adapted, are here inserted :

Medicines, with the Organs, etc., of the Body which they Specifically affect.

ACONITUM chiefly affects the circulating system.

ANTIMONIUM TART.—the pneumo-gastric nerve, the respiratory mucous membrane, and the skin.

ARNICA—the skin and absorbent vessels.

ARSENICUM chiefly affects the alimentary canal, respiratory organs, and skin.

BELLADONNA—the brain, nervous system generally, and the glands.

BRYONIA—the muscles, fibrous tissues of joints, lungs, respiratory organs, and liver.

CALCAREA—the mucous membranes, the fibrous system, the bones and skin.

CARBO VEGETABILIS—the organs of digestion.

CHAMOMILLA—the nervous system, liver, stomach, and bowels.

CINCHONA, or CHINA—the nervous system.

CINA—the stomach, intestinal canal, and brain.

COLOCYNTHIS—the stomach, bowels, brain, and nerves.

COFFEA—the whole nervous system.

CUPRUM—the cerebro-spinal and nervous system, and the abdominal viscera.

DROSERA—the bronchia.

DULCAMARA—the skin, mucous membranes, and glands.

HEPAR chiefly affects the glands, skin, mucous membranes, and windpipe.

IGNATIA—the brain and nervous system generally.

IPECACUANHA—the mucous membranes.

KALI BICHROMICUM—the mucous membranes, the glandular system (liver and kidneys), fibrous tissue, and skin.

MERCURIUS—the glands, skin, liver, and mucous membranes.

NUX VOMICA—the stomach, bowels, liver, and cerebral-spinal system.

PHOSPHORUS—the bronchia and respiratory organs.

PULSATILLA—the stomach, bowels, mucous membranes, and nervous system.

RHUS—the tendons, ligaments, and skin.

SPONGIA—the windpipe and bronchia.

SULPHUR—the skin, mucous membranes, and, to a great extent, the whole organism.

VERATRUM—the whole intestinal canal and brain.

Temperaments, Habits, and Conditions, with the Medicines peculiarly adapted to each.

Bilious Temperaments.—Aconitum, Bryonia, Chamomilla, Mercurius, Nux vomica, Pulsatilla.

Children or Infants.—Aconitum, Belladonna, Calcarea, Chamomilla, Ipecacuanha, Mercurius.

Debilitated Constitutions. — Arsenicum, Calcarea, Cinchona, Nux vomica, Sulphur, Kali bichromicum.

Females.—Aconitum, Belladonna, Chamomilla, Pulsatilla.

Females, Hysterical.—Ignatia, Nux vomica, Pulsatilla, Colocynthis.

Hypochondriachal Dispositions.—Calcarea, Nux vomica, Sulphur.

Nervous Temperament. — Aconitum, Chamomilla, Cinchona, Coffea, Ignatia, Nux vomica, Pulsatilla, Colocynthis.

Phlegmatic Temperament.—(Quiet, easy) Pulsatilla.

Plethoric Constitutions.—Aconitum, Belladonna, Nux vomica, Pulsatilla.

Sanguine Temperament. — Aconitum,

Materia Medica.

Arnica, Belladonna, Bryonia, Nux vomica.

Scrofulous Habit.—Arsenicum, Calca‑rea, Hepar, Mercurius, Sulphur.

INDEX.

Together with the Abbreviations of the Medicines most suited to each Complaint and Condition.

The DOSE, Page 13.

Index.

Index.

Index.

Index.

Index.

Index.

Index.

Index.

171

Index.

172

Index.

173

Index.

Index.

175

Index.

Index.

HOMŒOPATHIC BOOKS,

FOR

DOMESTIC PRACTICE.

SUITABLE FOR FAMILIES, TRAVELERS, AND STUDENTS.

PULTE'S Domestic Family Physician, $3.00
PULTE'S Woman's Medical Guide, - - 1.50
Popular Guide to Homœopathy, - - - 60

Douglas' Practical Homœopathy, . $0 75
Epps' Homœopathic Family Instructor, . 3 00
Ellis' Family Homœopathy, . . . 1 50
Freligh's Domestic, ... 3 50
Family Practice, or Simple Directions in
 Homœopathic Medicines, . . . 1 00
Guernsey's Domestic, ... 2 50
Hering's Domestic, ... 2 50
Hempel & Beakly's Theory and Practice, 3 50
Hempel's Domestic in German . . 75
Hempel's Domestic in French, . . . 75
Hill's Epitome. New Edition, . . 50
Hill's Epitome. In German, . . . 50
Laurie & M'Clatchey's Domestic Practice, 5 00
Morgan's Text-book for Domestic Practice, 60
Ruddock's Homœopathic Vade Mecum, . 3 00
Ruddock's Homœopathic Vade Mecum, extra
 bound, with Clinical Directory and article
 on Poisons, ... 5 00
Ruddock's Stepping-stone to Homœopathy
 and Health, ... 1 00
Ruddock's Ladies' Manual of Homœopathic
 Treatment of Diseases incident to her sex, 2 00
Shipman's Family Guide, . . . 1 50
Small's Domestic, ... 3 00
Tarbell's Homœopathy Simplified, . 1 25
The Sixteen Principal Homœopathic Remedies 1 00
Verdi on Maternity, a popular treatise for
 young wives and mothers, . . 2 25

www.ingramcontent.com/pod-product-compliance
Lightning Source LLC
Chambersburg PA
CBHW070927210326
41520CB00021B/6826